THE ACUPUNCTURE
TREATMENT OF PAIN

By the same author:

AMINO ACIDS IN THERAPY
CANDIDA ALBICANS
SOFT TISSUE MANIPULATION

THE ACUPUNCTURE TREATMENT OF PAIN

■

Safe and Effective Methods for Using Acupuncture in Pain Relief

▲

LEON CHAITOW

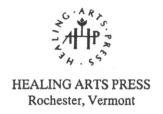

HEALING ARTS PRESS
Rochester, Vermont

Healing Arts Press
One Park Street
Rochester, Vermont 05767
www.innertraditions.com

Note to the reader: This book is intended as an informational guide. The remedies,
approaches, and techniques described herein are meant to supplement, and not
to be a substitute for, professional medical care or treatment. They should not
be used to treat a serious ailment without prior consultation
with a qualified healthcare professional.

LIBRARY OF CONGRESS CATALOGING-IN-PUBLICATION DATA
Chaitow, Leon.
The acupuncture treatment of pain.

Includes index.

1. Pain—Treatment. 2. Acupuncture. I. Title.
RB127.C45   1990   615.8'92   88-32007
ISBN 978-0-89281-383-4

Printed and bound in the United States

20 19 18 17 16 15 14 13 12 11

Healing Arts Press is a division of Inner Traditions International

CONTENTS

I dedicate this book to my parents,
Max and Irene,
with affection and gratitude

INTRODUCTION

In 1963 I attended the first English seminar on acupuncture, conducted by Dr J. Lavier of Paris. I was fascinated by the potential of the system but totally confused by the esoteric theories in which the system was cocooned. In the intervening years my studies have continued and I have come more and more to the view that the acupuncture phenomenon is scientifically explicable in terms acceptable to the Western mind. The purpose of this book is to tear away much of the mystique of acupuncture and to present to the healing profession a simple approach to pain relief, and the treatment of addiction.

I do not wish to suggest that acupuncture be confined to the relatively narrow limits of pain relief and addiction. Indeed, its usefulness in a great number of other diseases and conditions has been proved by many researchers, both in the West and in China. However, this book confines itself to the treatment of pain and the treatment of addiction, for which Western science has begun to offer scientifically acceptable explanations.

It is my hope that this work will be of use to all practitioners of the healing arts whether they be surgeons, general medical practitioners, osteopaths, chiropractors, physiotherapists, or trained nurses. I believe that anyone with the knowledge of anatomy and physiology required to join the ranks of these professions is capable of offering a great deal of relief to those in pain by using acupuncture. The methods are simple and safe if the rules are followed strictly.

Although acupuncture can be immensely useful, it has its limitations. We must be aware of these and not come to think of it as a cure-all. I find it a useful adjunctive system in my general approach to a patient, for unless it is combined with methods that remove causes, its results, though sometimes seemingly miraculous, are more often disappointing. In treating the symptoms of withdrawal from addiction this is equally true.

In describing the location of acupuncture points, I have given the Chinese name of the point together with the traditional meridian name and number, as well as a clear description of the anatomical position. On the page opposite each such description, an illustration will give further aid in the location of points.

Information as to the location of the more recently discovered points has been given as far as is possible. For example, the point on the auricle which influences the ankle will simply be called 'ankle point' (auricle) and reference should then be made to the illustration of the auricular points.

7

ACKNOWLEDGEMENTS

I wish to thank my illustator, Ken Morling, for his painstaking efforts. My grateful thanks also go to my wife, Alkmini, for her unstinting labour in typing and re-typing my notes, and her encouragement in my moments of doubt regarding this project.

1

Acupuncture for Pain Relief

Pain is the body's alarm signal, and when dealing with it, it is essential that the underlying causes are understood and that, where necessary, these are dealt with comprehensively. However, it is obviously desirable to relieve pain in the shortest possible space of time, and acupuncture offers a number of tried and tested formulae which can be utilized to this end, no matter which method is chosen by the practitioner to deal with the basic underlying causes.

Pain may be caused by any number of factors. To switch off a fire alarm and do nothing about the fire would be considered irresponsible, but there are times when, for some reason, the alarm goes off and does not stop ringing. Not long ago, in London, a man was prosecuted for climbing a ladder to an offending alarm bell (this not being the first time his peace had been disturbed) and wrenching it from its mounting. This action effectively cured his problem. The prosecution failed, for the court found that, all things considered, his action was justified.

In the same way, acupuncture can often switch off pain that has no useful role to play as a warning to the patient that all is not well. One example might be the neuritis that follows herpes zoster. I would suggest that before surgery was contemplated in such a condition as trigeminal neuralgia, an attempt should be made to ease the pain with acupuncture. If, however, pain is serving a useful purpose, we must think differently about controlling it. If a knee shows evidence of marked arthritic changes and it is considered that undue walking would increase the problem in the long term, then to simply ease the pain and do no more would be against the interests of the patient.

In such a case it might be that, in addition to pain control, the knee should be splinted to prevent too much movement, but whatever supplementary action is taken, the patient should be made to understand that the knee — though now hopefully relatively pain free — is not and cannot become normal, and should be used as little as possible. This is the contentious area in which pain control could fall into disrepute. Who would thank you for easing his pain whilst making him a cripple through lack of a comprehensive approach?

The majority of patients seek professional advice as a result of pain. In the following chapter we will examine some of the mechanisms involved in pain.

Palliative Treatment
Though simply using the symptomatic approach may produce no more than temporary improvement in chronic conditions where changes of a permanent nature have occurred in joints or other tissues, in certain acute conditions of recent onset — for example, traumatic torticollis or lumbosacral strains — the use of acupuncture symptomatically can in truth be a 'cure'. The relief of muscle spasm and the improvement in mobility may result in a speedy normalization of the painful condition.

9

At times, therefore, the easing of pain may be the desirable first step towards normalization and health. In some cases it is sufficient action in itself — the body's own efforts will do the rest. As we have seen, however, in the majority of cases the underlying causes of the condition must be dealt with. This might involve surgery, manipulation, dietetic changes, postural re-education, and so on, but whatever the final approach might be, the palliative nature of the initial pain control will have provided a more co-operative patient.

There is a tendency in many books on acupuncture to pour scorn on what are called 'second-class doctors' who provide palliative treatment. Indeed, this is acceptable criticism if a general approach to the patient's problem is thus avoided. It is not my suggestion that acupuncture should be so used. I sincerely wish to see a greater acceptance and use of acupuncture by all the healing professions. The simple methods and formulae set out in this book are not meant to cover the whole range of its possible uses in the treatment of disease, nor would I claim the book to be fully comprehensive regarding pain relief. It does, however, provide a broad base from which to start, and most areas of the body are dealt with from the particular viewpoint of pain control.

The fact that acupuncture is not (with obvious exceptions) an end in itself can be illustrated by considering its use to mask the pain of, say, advanced appendicitis, when the results could well be fatal. And if acupuncture were used to palliate any inflammatory joint disease, without other therapeutic measures being taken or the patient being properly advised as to limitations of activity, then such treatment could indeed be justifiably criticized. But in neither case would acupuncture be to blame. The dangerous use of an automobile by an irresponsible driver is no condemnation of the internal-combustion engine.

Traditional Philosophy of Acupuncture
The only other possible argument against the approach advocated in this book is that the practitioner should be completely versed in the whole philosophy of acupuncture in order to use it. This. however, is unnecessary. I maintain that much of what traditional acupuncturists hold to be true consists of theories and quaint explanations stemming from Chinese mythology and antiquity. The value of these to an age not versed in modern scientific terminology is obvious.

Myths and antique phraseology are often perpetuated as a result of an inability to see what is real in the vast literature that has grown around this subject during the thousands of years it has existed. Modern Chinese publications stress that until adequate explanations are forthcoming the old terminology will be used, but that this does not mean recognition of the myths and theories that surround such terminology. When I hear all this, I feel like the child in the story who yells the Emperor has no clothes — only in this case, whilst agreeing that the clothes are invisible, I would shout even more loudly that the Emperor does have teeth! Acupuncture works. But it works for sound physiological reasons through the neuro-endocrine system, not because of an interplay of Yin and Yang, however attractive such a metaphysical hypothesis might seem.

10

A Basic Set of Rules

The rules are simple, but must be followed strictly in order to obtain results and, more importantly, in order to maintain the safety of the patient. It is no more necessary to understand the workings of the engine of a car in order to drive it than it is to understand fully the way acupuncture works, in order to use it. In both cases, however, a basic set of rules must be adhered to in order to prevent disasters.

Some people argue that before using acupuncture the practitioner should memorize all the points on the surface of the body. There are more than 1000 of these points. Over the centuries, the myriad reflex effects of many of these have been defined, and the theories and explanations for the effects of massaging or needling particular points and groups of points have evolved. It is these theories and beliefs that have become the fabric of acupuncture (and, I believe, the fabric of the Emperor's non-existent clothes!).

It is possible to demonstrate particular effects following acupuncture treatment. Some of these effects involve the alteration of the function of organs or systems. There is an analgesic effect and also an anaesthetic effect. The reflexes involved may not yet be fully explained, but if we cling to the archaic explanations, however colourful and attractive they sound, we will never uncover the full potential of this system. Is it necessary to hold that imbalance between Yin and Yang (the two equal and opposite forces of the universe which act through Chi) is the cause of disease? Is it not more reasonable to talk in terms of the body's homeostatic tendency, whereby a stable internal environment is maintained through the interaction of the various body processes and systems? Those modern acupuncturists who cling to traditional phraseology do a disservice to their science. In China, acupuncture was used in combination with herbal medicine, dietetic regimes and psychological guidance. In the same way, we should use it as an adjunct to a broad approach to the patient and his problems. The memorizing of all the points on the body is not necessary for the successful application of acupuncture techniques. It is sufficient to know the rules and to follow them precisely — points can be looked up as and when they are needed.

2

How Does Acupuncture Work?

My wife is Greek and through her I have come to know and love Greece and its heritage. My love for the spiritual beauty represented by icons leads me to an important thought in my attempt to explain my apparent antipathy towards the semantics of traditional acupuncture. Icons were first used by the church to illustrate intangible ideas and spiritual thoughts. As time went by, the icons themselves tended to become the objects of worship and this led to iconoclasm — a desire on behalf of reformers to destroy the images, not because of what they were but because of what they had been used for. I love the beauty of icons but they are not God and should I start to ascribe to them the power that is God's then it would be better to burn them rather than to continue in idolatry. I love the poetic language and the beautiful harmony of traditional acupuncture theories, but they do not assist in my understanding of the true nature of health and disease and so must be set aside.

An example of this is the pulse-taking technique which is a major part of traditional acupuncture. Dr George Lewith[1] describes it thus:

> The palpation of the pulse enables the acupuncturist to assess which organ is diseased, whether the organ is over- or under-active, and the pathogen causing the damage. This is achieved by feeling the pulse at three positions at each wrist, and by feeling the pulse at the superficial and deep positions at each end of three positions on the wrist. There are six pulses at each wrist, three superficial and three deep. There are twelve main organs in the Chinese medical system and each of these is represented by one of the pulses at one of the wrist positions. . . . This method of diagnosis allows the whole body to be assessed, and it also defines the relative balance between each of the organs.

The enormity of the suspension of critical judgement that such a system calls for is hinted at by Lewith when he says:

> The observation that each of these pulses represents a different organ is a difficult fact to accept and understand. It is astonishing to think that different organs are represented by the pulse in the left and right hands, and that these pulses are separated only by a centimetre or so.

Louise Wensel, also a medical practitioner, comes closer to my viewpoint when, after describing the system in some detail, she states:[2]

> The traditional acupuncturist is concerned with these reciprocal interactions. Since all these 'pulses' are on the radial artery, however, near the same position where Americans and Europeans usually check a patient's pulse, it seems strange and misleading to consider them as separate, and it is no longer considered necessary for an acupuncturist to learn pulse diagnosis.

It would seem that there is, amongst Western trained Acupuncturists, a tendency therefore to pay lip-service to some aspects of the traditional methodology of acupuncture, whilst at the same time discreetly abandoning their use.

[1] *Acupuncture: Its Place in Western Medical Science* by George T. Lewith M.A., M.R.C.G.P., M.R.C.P. (Thorsons, 1982).
[2] *Acupuncture in Medical Practice* by Louise Wensel (Reston Publishing Co. Inc., 1980).

This trend coincides with discoveries and developments in the West which begin to explain some of the mechanisms by which acupuncture achieves its results. It is in modern scientific terms that we must seek explanations and not attempt to marry the classical interpretations, which were based on philosophical concepts rather than on facts, with physiological evidence which points in other directions. Some do attempt this syntheses. David Bresler Ph.D. in his contribution to *Health for the Whole Person*[3] states:

> Do all of these scientific findings mean that the traditional theory of energy flow has no practical validity? The answer to this depends upon the perspective of the questioner. Modern physics has shown that matter and energy are not distinct but represent two aspects of the same thing. In some situations, it is easier to explain a given phenomenon in terms of matter; in others, in terms of energy. Likewise, all events in the organism, whether psychological or physiological, involve both matter and energy. Thus, it does not seem at all contradictory to think both in terms of energy flow and of physiological mechanisms, in order to explain what is happening when acupuncture is performed.

This may be satisfactory on a theoretical level. In practical terms I find the physiological explanation more helpful.

We are on shaky ground if we start to translate old theories into modern terms. In many old texts, different qualities were ascribed to needles made of different metals such as silver and gold. It can be demonstrated that this is not only untrue, but that needles themselves are not essential to the performance of acupuncture. Indeed, electrical stimulation or digital pressure is often sufficient stimulus to produce the desired effect. So the pitfall of granting to the needles any magical power must be avoided. The body heals itself. The needles or pressure or electrical impulses provide the body with a stimulus and the body itself responds to this.

For many years osteopaths and chiropractors have used reflex pressure techniques to assist the body in its efforts towards health. Many of the points used correspond with acupuncture points.

If it is accepted that the body will constantly strive towards health, then it must be agreed that it will use all helpful stimuli to that end, If, through acupuncture or manual pressure, this function can be assisted, the homeostatic interplay of organ systems will carry on the work to the extent possible at that time.

Responses to Stimuli

How are stimuli received and handled by the body? Is it via a hypothetical flow of energy on the body's surface? Is it by triggering chemical changes in the area of the needle insertion? Is it by means of neuro-endocrine stimulation via normal neural pathways? Is it by 'confusing' the brain into rejecting pain stimuli? Or is it not possible that different effects have different *modus operandi*? Pain relief might well be the result of neurally mediated changes in the brain's receptivity to pain impulses, as well as an effect of biochemical changes due to the release of hormone-like substances both locally and generally.

[3] *Health for the Whole Person* by A. C. Hastings Ph.D., J. Fadiman Ph.D. and J. Gordon M.D. (Westview Press, 1981).

How does acupuncture work? In considering this for the purpose of pain relief, we are more concerned with how it can be used as an analgesic and anaesthetic than with the other effects and their possible mechanism although certain hypotheses will be examined in an effort to shed light on the subject.

According to the Peking Acupuncture Anaesthesia Co-ordinating Group,[4] research using ECG readings shows that acupuncture analgesia and anaesthesia are a result of activity within the cerebral cortex and various sub-cortical levels of the central nervous system (with possible participation of other factors, i.e. humoral). They quote widespread evidence (over 400,000 operations under acupuncture anaesthesia up to 1970) to prove that needling or *pressing* certain points is effective in stopping pain in remote body areas.

The body is able to use stimuli to its own best advantage.

The same Peking group states that stimulation of one point will assist correction of both high and low blood-pressure, a further point will bring a rapid or slow heart rate towards normal, and further points will increase the number of white blood corpuscles and intensify phagocytosis. These regulating effects must surely result from neuro-endocrine responses.

More recent research[5] demonstrated that vascular occlusion of the upper arm could not prevent the analgesic effect of acupuncture of a point on the hand from being mediated to other regions of the body as manifested by the raising of pain thresholds at those regions. It was also shown that infiltration of procaine in the deep tissues around the acupuncture point abolished entirely the distant analgesic effect. This suggested to the researchers of the Shanghai Institutes of Physiology and Traumatology that the nervous system, and not humoral activity, was responsible for the mediation of the analgesic effect.

Bilateral Analgesic Effects
A further result of the research was to show that the stimulation of a point had bilateral analgesic effects. Thus in knee surgery it was possible to use points on the healthy leg to anaesthetize the opposite leg. This important research claims that there exists a segmental relationship between the needled point and the area of analgesia.

A recently published report by the Shanghai Acupuncture Anaesthesia Co-ordinating Group[6] shows that afferent impulses for acupuncture analgesia were transmitted mainly via the deep nerves which innervate the deep fascia, tendinous sheaths, muscles, periostia, etc. It was also demonstrated that acupuncture was able to excite different sensory receptors, such as tension and pressure receptors, in the deep tissues.

After complex investigation they inferred that the afferent pathways of the acupuncture effect were closely related to those of pain and temperature

[4] *Acupuncture Anaesthesia,* Foreign Language Press, Peking, 1972.
[5] *Scienta Sinica,* Vol. XVI, No. 2, page 210, Science Press, Peking, 1973.
[6] *Chinese Medical Journal,* January 1975, page 13.

sensations in the spinal cord, whilst the persistence of the effect was more or less related to the pathways for proprioceptive sensations. In order to illustrate the role of the integrative action of the thalamus in the process of acupuncture analgesia, potential changes in single nerve cells in the thalamus were recorded with microelectrodes and subjected to analysis. Results indicate that the degree of efficacy of acupuncture analgesia might be influenced to a large extent by the state of brain excitability of the subject.

A further series of experiments, in which the cephalic ends of the carotid arteries of two animals were cross-connected, indicated that humoral factors do participate in the acupuncture effect. Pain thresholds were elevated in one animal by acupuncture stimulation of the other.

Finger-pressure Acupuncture
Another series of animal experiments was conducted by the research group at Peking Medical College.[7] It was found that needle stimulation of (Tsu) San Li (Stomach point 36) produced a rise of 128 per cent in the pain threshold, which lasted for forty minutes. Finger-pressure stimulation of Kun Lun (Bladder point 60) produced a rise of 133 per cent.

The research group stated that, on human subjects, needle acupuncture did not always produce the aimed-for sensation. On many occasions, the direction and depth of needling, and the amplitude of twisting of the needle, had to be adjusted according to the feelings of the individual undergoing treatment. They found, however, that the use of finger-pressure acupuncture could successfully induce the desired feeling of soreness and fullness that is a forerunner of the anaesthetic effect. Electrophysiological studies showed that deep pressure applied to muscles and tendons had a definite inhibitory effect on the unit discharge of neurons in the non-specific nucleus of the thalamus.

During the course of animal experiments (in this case, rabbits) artificial cerebro-spinal fluid was perfused through the animal receiving finger-pressure acupuncture. When this perfusate was drawn off and injected into the ventricle of a recipient rabbit, the latter showed a pain threshold rise of eighty-two per cent. Those experiments were performed using controls, and the difference between experimental and control animals was highly significant, indicating the presence of some chemical substance or substances with analgesic effects in the CSF following acupuncture. The more recent knowledge of endorphins (for example) helps to explain many of these results.

These and many other experiments using animals indicate that the analgesic effect of acupuncture is not related to any hypnotic effect or to psychological suggestibility on the part of the patient.

It is well known that the mental state of the patient will exercise certain influences on his reaction to sensory stimuli. If he is in good spirits and co-operative, the effects of acupuncture treatment to raise pain thresholds will be more

[7] *Scienta Sinica,* Vol. XVII, No. 1, page 112, Science Press, Peking, 1974.

successful than in an uncooperative and nervous individual. However, the patient's subjective initiative cannot replace the acupuncture anaesthesia; the physiological and psychological factors are interrelated and one promotes the other.

Neuro-humoral Mechanisms?
If we remove from the acupuncture phenomenon the concepts of Yin and Yang, and of 'Vital energy' or 'life force', what are we left with? Certainly we cannot claim that neuro-anatomy and neuro-physiology can as yet provide a full answer. I would contend, however, that sufficient evidence has been garnered to point towards the acupuncture effect being explained by neuro-humoral mechanisms. The degree of research and investigation into those aspects, as yet unexplained by modern scientific knowledge, is in itself a tribute to the clinical genius of the traditional acupuncture practitioners. Their theories may not stand up to modern investigations but they have certainly pushed forward the understanding of physiology as we knew it.

But several unanswered questions remain. What, for example, is the connection between the auricular surface and distant areas and organs? That there is some such connection is demonstrable.[8] A variety of experiments have been conducted to give clear cut evidence to this end.

In one such[9], after insertion of needles into four ear points, pain sensitivity was assessed by probing the abdominal wall at regular intervals with a needle. The first test was done after five minutes, followed each minute thereafter for fifteen minutes. There was progressive reduction in the intensity of pain, from sharp to dull, and by the final needle probe, no pain at all. The induction time here is significant, since failure to achieve results often follows too hasty removal of needles from the ear.

William Lowe M.D.[10] points out that the ear has an abundant innervation being supplied by the sensory fibres of the trigeminal, fascial and vagus nerves and the greater auricular and greater and lesser occipital nerves. The endings of these nerves are closely interwoven and superimposed, providing access through them to influence many distant body areas.

The efficacy of ear acupuncture is well established and it is only a matter of time before full understanding of its modus operandi is forthcoming. For a deeper understanding of the subject it is suggested that study be made of the work of Dr Paul Nogier[11]. There is some discrepancy between Nogier's location of points and the Chinese locations. This highlights the need to seek, and probe, for sensitivity in

[8]*Scienta Sinica,* Vol. XVI, No. 3, page 455, Science Press, Peking, 1973.
[9]S. Chiang. 'Ear Needles for Acupuncture Anaesthesia' — *Liberation Daily News,* 5 January 1972.
[10]*Introduction to Acupuncture Anaesthesia,* by W. C. Lowe M.D. (Medical Examination Pub. Co. N.Y., 1973).
[11]*Treatise on Auriculotherapy,* by Paul F. Nogier (Maisonneuve, 1972).

points prior to needling. There is evidence[12] that some points produce a specific localized effect and others (such as Ho-Ku, LI4) produce generalized analgesic or anaesthetic effects throughout the body. Combining a specific and a general effect point (if they palpate as sensitive and/or produce a low reading in terms of electrical resistance) would seem to produce the best results, in terms of pain relief.

Western research has so far produced no great breakthrough in our understanding of acupuncture. The theory of a 'gate' in the substantia gelatinosa in the dorsal horn of the spinal cord was put forward by Meljack (McGill University) and Wall (University College, London). This 'gate', which closes itself to pain stimuli upon receipt of the milder stimulation of the acupuncture needle, was elaborated into a 'two-gate' theory by Cheu and Man,[13] in which the thalamus was claimed to be a second gate. The recent discovery of endogenous polypeptides which link to opiate receptors in the brain and central nervous system offers a new vista to the acupuncture phenomenon. It seems certain that the analgesic effect of acupuncture is to some extent mediated by the release of these endorphins (*endogenous morphines*). This is further discussed in the chapter on the treatment of addiction.

Electrical Resistance

A further aspect of the acupuncture phenomenon is that the acupuncture points on the body's surface are demonstrably areas of lower electrical resistance. Equipment which measures the electrical impedance of the skin was developed in France by Dr Niboyet before the last war. This has been elaborated on over the years, and in Western Europe has led to a discarding of the meridian theory and the evolvement of the idea of pathways of neuro-electrical impulses working through the autonomic nervous system.

A more recent step in this direction was taken by the Japanese researcher, Dr Nakatani,[14] who states that the excitability of the sympathetic nerves of the skin may be measured through variations in the electrical resistance of specific points. These points, which in many instances correlate exactly with traditional acupuncture points, are used for both diagnosis and treatment of functional diseases and of pain. The system which developed from research in Japan is known as Ryodoraku acupuncture therapy. The theory postulates that when abnormalities exist in internal organs or when the function of an organ changes, there are corresponding changes on the surface. These may result from sensory nerve reflexes, motor nerve reflexes, and sympathetic or parasympathetic nerve reflexes. Dr Nakatani states that he believes that the local skin point, which is peripheral to the autonomic nervous system, may act as a synapse where localized hormones are secreted and that there is a two-way feedback along the sympathetic nerve, thus allowing both diagnosis and treatment from the same point.

[12]C. Hsing. 'Specificity and non specificity of Acupuncture Points — *Liberation Daily News,* 23 December 1971.
[13]Current Therapy Researches 14 (No. 7), July 1972.
[14]Gunji, *Introduction to Simple Ryodoraku Treatment,* Bunkodo Co. Ltd., Tokyo, 1971.

Acupuncture and Osteopathy

There is a correlation between acupuncture point networks and osteopathic musculoskeletal lesion patterns. According to Regard,[15] one system proves the validity of the other in diagnostic and therapeutic application. According to Dr Nemerhof,[16] neither method considers itself to be an independent or exclusive healing art for patient care; but both systems employ neuro-mechanical forms of therapy to restore homeostasis to the body.

Dr Felix Mann,[17] in discussing the bladder meridian (part of which is paravertebral), speaks of acupuncture as being 'Chinese Osteopathy'.

Nemerhof[15] points out that in modern terms acupuncture theory is based on the inter-connection of acupuncture points with the autonomic nervous system network. He confirms the opinion of Regard that acupuncture in conjunction with osteopathic manipulative techniques is effective treatment in managing conditions of chronic trauma. Nemerhof makes the important point that neither acupuncture nor osteopathy provides a final answer to complete patient management, but that, applied appropriately, acupuncture can amplify the possibilities of patient cure.

Dr A. Becker[18] has compared the central nervous system to a digital computer and the mind to an analogue computer, and he hypothesizes that the effectiveness of acupuncture might be explained by visualizing the insertion of needles as a means of selectively shorting a circuit through which the computer normally carries out a specific function. This he compares with flicking an enabling (or disabling) switch which bypasses certain functions of the computer without stopping its operation in other ways.

Acupuncture can be seen to be a useful, physiologically-based tool in the hands of the healing professions.

When we scratch an itch or rub a sore area we are instinctively attempting to substitute one set of messages to the brain with other more acceptable messages. For every action there is a reaction, and the body will respond to stimuli on various levels. Much depends on the site, duration and nature of the stimulus. It is precisely the site, duration and nature (needle, pressure or electrical stimulation) which determine whether we are to achieve stimulation, sedation or anaesthesia.

Traditionalists maintain that energy (*Chi*) is being 'supplied' or drained away. Mary Austin[19] suggests that it is essential when 'draining' a painful area that 'vital energy' be replaced by stimulating either Ho Ku (Large Intestine point 4) or Kun Lun (Bladder point 60). There may well prove to be physiological reasons for this empirical traditional approach. However, I contend that, if current research is to be

[15]P. Regard, *Proceedings of Third International Congress of Physical Medicine,* Westlake Press, Chicago, 1962.
[16]*Journal of the American Osteopathic Association,* December 1972, page 346/51.
[17]F. Mann, *Acupuncture, The Ancient Chinese Art of Healing,* Heinemann Medical Books.
[18]'Parameters of Resistance', *Journal of the American Osteopathic Association,* September 1973, page 39/75.
[19]Mary Austin, *Acupuncture Therapy,* Turnstone Press, 1974.

trusted, the explanation that 'vital energy' is being replaced will be found to be incorrect.

The Body's Response

It is important to keep in mind that the really vital factor in treatment is the response of the body. It is not the needle but the nature of the response to the needle that counts.

Simple insertion of a needle (or momentary deep pressure) acts as a stimulant. Left *in situ* for five to twenty minutes, the needle (or sustained pressure) has a sedating, numbing effect on local or remote (reflex) tissues. If this were to continue, then the anaesthetic effect would become apparent. These responses are physiological. Any stimulant, be it alcohol or cold water, would have similarly contradictory effects. Try to compare the difference between the body's response to a half-minute cold bath and half an hour in cold water; or compare the consumption of a tot of whisky with half a bottle of whisky!

Much more research will be done and results will no doubt alter views now generally held, but it is within accepted physiological frameworks that explanations will be found.

In his study of the nature of disease, Speransky[20] explained how, after years of research, he became convinced that, in studying the processes of disease, the traditional subdivision of the nervous system into central, peripheral, sympathetic, etc. had no justification. He showed in many experiments that, from any point in the nervous system, it was possible to bring into action nerve mechanisms, the functioning of which terminated at the periphery, producing changes of a bio-physico-chemical character.

He developed the thesis that any nerve point, not excluding peripheral nerve structures, could become the originator of neuro-dystrophic processes serving as the temporary or permanent nerve centre of these processes, and pointed out that whenever a procedure affected the nervous aspect of any phenomenon, the resultant changes were not only in the nerve portion concerned, but *in the whole intricate complex. Also apparent from his work was the fact that irritation of any point of the nervous system could evoke changes, not only in the adjacent parts, but also in remote regions of the organism.*

Finally, he stated that it became evident that the usefulness of operating on the nervous system was often due to the very act of interference itself and not to its form, whilst harm depended on its form and was associated with excessive trauma. I find in these thoughts of Speransky's the justification for my views on acupuncture and, in a large part, the explanation for the acupuncture phenomenon.

Added to this, the new knowledge of endorphins and enkephalines provide at least the basis for accepting that there are physiological reasons for acupuncture's results. Whatever the psychological factors which are concurrently at work it is clear that beneficial biochemical changes, probably neurally mediated (at least in part) are at work.

[20]A. Speransky, *A Basis for the Theory of Medicine,* International Publishers, New York, 1943.

19

3

How to Use Acupuncture

Needles

Modern acupuncture needles tend to be made of stainless steel with a handle of copper or aluminium. They must be sufficiently flexible to avoid the breakage which may occur due to muscle spasm after insertion. The handle is important in both the insertion and subsequent manipulation of the needle. The length of the needle varies from half an inch to five inches and in thickness from twenty-six gauge to thirty-two gauge. Many practitioners use standard disposable thirty-gauge hypodermic needles. The shorter needles are used in superficial areas such as the head and face, and the longer ones in the fleshier regions. An indication of the required depth of insertion will be given with each formula point, but variations will occur in different body types, and the practitioner's own judgement should be used. Often a sensation of fullness or radiating warmth will be felt by the patient when a needle reaches the desired depth. Although this is not essential for good results, it often seems to accompany the more successful applications of acupuncture.

Aseptic procedures are desirable in acupuncture. Needles should be sterile and both the area of insertion and the hands of the practitioner should be prepared as for parenteral injection. Immediately prior to insertion, the site and the sterile needle should be wiped with alcohol or an antiseptic swab. Needles should be examined for defects before use, and if they are bent or if the point is not pefectly sharp they should be discarded.

Care must be taken in treating vertebral points, as insertion of a needle into the central nervous system could produce transient paralysis. All such problems will be avoided if the points used correspond exactly with those recommended and the depth of insertion does not exceed that advised in the text.

Location and Selection of Points

In order to accurately locate acupuncture points we use two systems of description. One is the description of the exact anatomical position and this is obviously the simplest method. However, there are many points which do not fall into exact locations and whose individual location depends upon the dimensions of the patient. In order to take account of variations in body size, the Chinese developed the 'human inch' or 'cun'. We will call this unit of measurement, which not only differs from patient to patient, but from one body area to another, the Acupuncture Unit of Measurement (AUM). The AUM of the forearm, for example, is determined by measuring the distance between the wrist crease and the cubital crease, and dividing by twelve.

A full list of proportional measurements is as follows.

The AUM of the head is calculated by one of the following measurements: midline of the anterior hairline to midline of the posterior hairline, which equals 12 AUM; the distance between the anterior hairline and the glabella, which is 3 AUM;

and the distance between the posterior hairline and the seventh cervical spinous process, which is 3 AUM (if the hairline is indistinguishable, then the distance from the glabella to the spinous process of the seventh cervical vertebrae is 18 AUM).

The AUM of the back is calculated by measuring the distance from the midline to the medial border of the scapula, which is 3 AUM. The AUM of the thorax and abdomen is calculated by measuring the distance between the nipples — 8 AUM. The lower end of the sternum to the umbilicus is also 8 AUM. From the umbilicus to the upper border of the symphasis pubis is 5 AUM.

The AUM of the upper arm is calculated by measuring from the axillary fold to the cubital elbow crease, a distance of 9 AUM.

The AUM for the upper leg is calculated by measuring from the proximal point of the greater trochanter to the lower aspect of the patella — 19 AUM.[1] The AUM of the lower leg is calculated by measuring either the distance from the middle of the patella to the prominence of the lateral malleolus, which is 16 AUM, or the distance from the medial condyle of the tibia to the prominence of the medial malleolus, which is 13 AUM.

Another method of measuring the dimension of the patient's AUM is to use the finger length of the patient in the following manner: the distance between the two creases of the interphalangeal joints of the patient's middle finger, when flexed, represents 1 AUM. A further guide is that the width of the patient's four fingers represents 3 AUM.

These techniques are fairly accurate and, when combined with anatomical descriptions of location, should provide the practitioner with sufficient information to locate specific points accurately.

The Meridians

The patterns which acupuncture points make on the body's surface have been charted by practitioners of acupuncture for centuries. They have been grouped together in lines (called channels or meridians) and have been allocated to the organs or functions upon which they appear to act. In addition to the twelve pairs of bilateral meridians, there are two meridians which lie on the anterior and posterior midline of the trunk and head, and there also exist various extra-meridians which link the fourteen meridians. Apart from these patterns of acupuncture points which appear to relate to the body's organs and functions, there are other points in the ear surfaces, the hands and the face which have specific reflex effects. Clinically, there is abundant evidence to indicate the existence of reflex links between acupuncture points and specific organs and functions.

From the viewpoint of pain relief it is useful to know the patterns and pathways of the meridians. The usefulness of such knowledge occurs in the selection of points which are some distance from a site of pain, where the only apparent relationship is via such a meridian pathway. The theory that energy flows along these pathways and that disease results from an excess or deficiency of energy in the meridians has

[1] Many texts published in the West give this distance as 13 AUM. This book follows the modern Chinese measurement.

not been substantiated. What is valid is the clinical experience that has created the knowledge of the reflex effects of acupuncture points and the interrelationships that exist between the various pathways.

Distant Points
The usefulness of treating points distant from a site of pain has been clinically proved. In certain rheumatic and muscular conditions, distant points may be treated prior to local points being used. During treatment the patient may be instructed to exercise or move the affected area. Indications as to where such techniques may prove helpful will be given in the formulary. In the treatment of such conditions as headaches or trigeminal neuralgia, it is often a good idea to use distant points on a meridian that contains local points in the area of pain. In the treatment of post-herpes neuritis, for example, a knowledge of the pathways of the various meridians is a help in the selection of distant points for treatment. Information will be given in the formulary as to which distant points may be used in the treatment of various painful conditions.

It is important to grasp the true nature of the meridians. In a recent book on acupuncture,[2] the Academy of Traditional Chinese Acupuncture states: 'The ancients discovered, in the course of struggling against disease, that stimulating certain spots of the body surface ameliorated internal diseases. They called such "spots" points. They further discovered that stimulating a definite series of points ameliorated the syndrome of diseases of a specific organ. As they connected these points and the functions of the organs into a system, the theory of the channels and collaterals (extra-meridians) was gradually formed. *However, owing to the restrictions placed by existing social conditions and the limited scientific knowledge it was impossible then to further research into this theory.'* (My italics.)

The book goes on: 'Personnel of both Chinese and Western medicine are doing a great deal of research in the theory of channels (meridians). They have come to the conclusion that the channels are closely related to the nerves, blood vessels and body fluids.'

Thus the home of acupuncture appears to reject the traditional theory of a flow of 'vital energy' through the channels (meridians). Reflex pathways which relate to organs and functions of the body do exist. Points on these pathways are reflexly linked to each other.

There exist a number of machines that can further assist in the location of points. Such equipment measures the electrical resistance of the skin surface and provides either visual or audible confirmation of the location of the points required.

Guidelines in Choosing Points
In using the formulae given in this book, it is suggested that points be chosen for use according to the following guidelines.

The points selected may be chosen so that they encircle the area of pain. If this is

[2] *An Outline of Chinese Acupuncture,* Foreign Language Press, Peking, 1975.

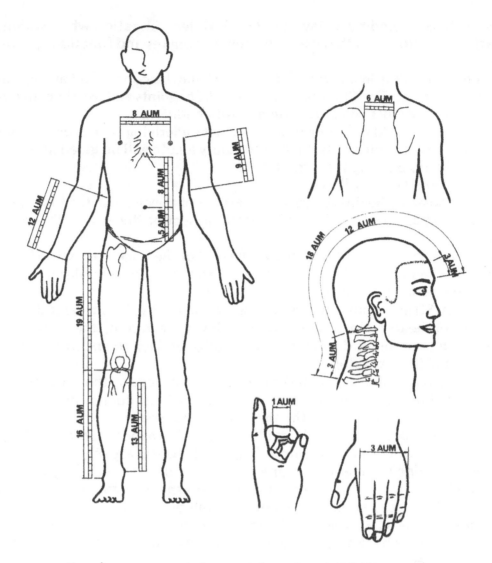

Shows proportional measurements to ascertain patients' AUM (Acupuncture Units of Measurement) in different body areas.

not possible, a line of points on a limb may be treated. But in addition to using local points, it will be found that the formulae often contain points that are distant from the site of pain, and these may be combined with local points. It must be remembered that there is a contralateral effect in acupuncture and good results can be obtained by choosing points accordingly. Thus in treating pain in the right elbow, suitable points may be chosen on both arms in order to reinforce the analgesic effect. It should be remembered that if an area is swollen or inflamed, acupuncture needles must not be placed directly into the site, but should be inserted into the nearest suitable points.

Modern research indicates that the meridians are autonomic fibres in which the energy cycle is altered by a wave of electrical depolarization when stimulated.[3] The various relationships that exist with specific organs and functions are reflex in nature.

Local tender points in an area of discomfort may be considered as spontaneous acupuncture points. The Chinese term these *Ah Shi* points and use them in the same way as classical points when treating painful conditions.

Practitioners should ascertain precisely what underlying tissues exist in deciding upon treatment of such points. In the formulary a note will be given as to when *Ah Shi* points should be sought for treatment.

The meridians are as follows:

The lung meridian (L) begins on the lateral aspect of the chest, in the first intercostal space. It then passes down the anterolateral aspect of the arm to the root of the thumbnail.

The large intestine (LI) meridian starts at the root of the fingernail of the first finger. It passes up the posterolateral aspect of the arm over the shoulder to the face. It ends at the side of the nostril.

The stomach (St) meridian starts below the orbital cavity, It runs over the face and up to the forehead from where it passes down the throat, the thorax and the abdomen, and continues down the anterior thigh and leg to end at the root of the second toenail (lateral side).

The spleen (Sp) meridian originates at the medial aspect of the great toe. It then travels up the internal aspect of the leg and thigh to the abdomen and thorax, where it finishes on the axillary line in the sixth intercostal space.

The heart (H) meridian begins in the axilla and runs down the anteromedial aspect of the arm to end at the root of the little fingernail (medial aspect).

The small intestine (Si) meridian starts at the root of the small fingernail (lateral aspect) and then travels up the posteromedial aspect of the arm, and over the shoulder to the face, where it terminates in front of the ear.

The bladder (B) meridian starts at the inner canthus, ascends and passes over the head, and down the back and the leg, to terminate at the root of the nail of the little toe (lateral aspect).

The kidney (K) meridian starts on the sole of the foot. It ascends the medial aspect of the leg and runs up the front of the abdomen to finish on the thorax, just below the clavicle.

The circulation (C) meridian (also known as heart constrictor or pericardium) begins on the thorax lateral to the nipple. It runs down the anterior surface of the arm and terminates at the root of the nail of the middle finger.

The triple-heater (TH) meridian begins at the nail root of the ring finger (ulna side) and runs up the posterior aspect of the arm, over the back of the shoulder and around the ear to finish at the outer aspect of the eyebrow.

The gall bladder (GB) meridian starts at the outer canthus and runs backwards and forwards over the head, passing over the front of the shoulder, and down the lateral

[3] F. Mann, *Meridians of Acupuncture,* Heinemann Medical Books, 1971.

aspect of the thorax and abdomen. It passes to the hip area and thence down the lateral aspect of the leg to terminate on the fourth toe.

The liver (Liv) meridian begins on the great toe, runs up the medial aspect of the leg, up the abdomen, and terminates on the costal margin (vertically below the nipple).

The foregoing are all bilateral, symmetrically distributed lines of acupuncture points with affinity for or effects upon the functions or organs for which they are named.

There are two midline meridians, the *Conception Vessel* (CV) meridian starts in the centre of the perineum, and runs up the midline of the anterior aspect of the body to terminate just below the lower lip; the *Governor Vessel* (GV) meridian starts at the coccyx and runs up the centre of the spine, over the midline of the head, and terminates on the front of the upper gum.

Needle Insertion and Manipulation

Both the needle and the skin area surrounding the point to be treated should be wiped with an antiseptic solution. The patient should be recumbent and relaxed prior to treatment. For the insertion of relatively short needles, the following method should be followed.

Pressure is applied with the finger or the thumb of the left hand (nail pressure may be used) to the area immediately next to the site of insertion. At the same time the needle, which should be held by its handle between the forefinger and the thumb of the right hand, is inserted and twisted. There may be transient pain as the needle breaks the skin, but thereafter only a sensation of fullness or of radiating warmth should be felt.

Longer needles may also be held by the stem so that a controlled, speedy penetration of the skin is achieved; while the left hand stabilizes the stem of the needle, a combined rotation and pressure by the right hand on the handle will guide it to the desired depth. On areas where there is little muscle (e.g. the face), the skin around the point may be pinched gently by the fingers of the left hand whilst insertion is made. On areas where tissues are loose or where there are creases or folds of skin, such as the abdomen, the skin may be stretched prior to insertion.

A further technique for insertion is to use fine needles that can pass through a narrow metal, glass or plastic tube (such as a drinking straw). The tube is placed over the point and the needle is rested in it with its handle protruding slightly. A firm tap will send the needle through the skin, and by swiftly removing the tube the needle may then be guided and rotated to its desired depth. This method is less painful to the patient but the precise point of entry may not be so accurate.

The direction of insertion may be perpendicular, oblique or horizontal. In the main muscular areas of the body, where a deep insertion is required, perpendicular insertions will normally be used. If an oblique insertion is required, the angle will usually be between thirty and forty-five degrees. A horizontal insertion will usually only be required on the head or face.

Unless otherwise stated in the formulary, insertions suggested therein will be perpendicular. The depth of insertion will depend to a large extent on the body type of the patient and this should be considered when deciding on the degree of penetration required. Guidance will be given in the text as to the depth of penetration required. A sensation of fullness, heaviness and tingling may be experienced when the needle reaches its desired depth. In treating auricular points, a short (half-inch) needle should be used. Insertion should be through the skin and into the cartilage. Manipulation of the needle is then performed in the same way as in other body areas. Lavier[4] states that in order to achieve sedation the needle insertion must be swift and the withdrawal slow. This is confirmed by Chu-Lien.[5]

In the treatment of pain I have found that periodic rotation of the needle, combined with a degree of lifting and thrusting, assists the analgesic effect. This may be repeated every few minutes for up to half an hour. Constant manipulation appears to be necessary in order to achieve an anaesthetic effect and this is best achieved by electrical stimulation of the needle (see Chapter 7). In treating chronic conditions, the needles should be left *in situ* for up to thirty minutes. Acute conditions may require longer, but fifteen to thirty minutes twice daily should produce relief. A course of treatment in a chronic condition would consist of fifteen to twenty treatments with two or three days between treatments. After this, treatment should not be resumed for several weeks.

Moxibustion
The application of heat to the acupuncture point is known as moxibustion. For the treatment of pain, I recommend the technique of indirect heating, in which a small piece of moxa (dried leaves of *Artemesia vulgaris*) is placed on the inserted needle handle and is then ignited. The heat is conducted to the deep tissues through the needle. There are points on which moxibustion is forbidden and due regard should be taken of this when using the formulae. The notes relating to the treatment of a particular area will indicate whether this technique is recommended or forbidden. The symbol △ on any chart or drawing of acupuncture points indicates that moxibustion should not be performed on that point. (Note that some points are suitable for moxibustion but not for needle insertion. Moxibustion is then performed by direct application of a small cone of moxa to the skin surface. Such points are indicated on charts by the symbol □.)

The removal of the needle should take place when it is not being 'gripped' by the tissues in which it lies. If it has become bent through muscular spasm, removal must be slow and gentle. Never force the needle to withdraw, even if it means leaving it in position for some time. Gently massage the area or rotate the needles slowly to aid the relaxation of the tissues.

As I have mentioned earlier, it is quite possible to use acupuncture without a needle. The response of the body to the manual pressure of acupuncture points is the same as that achieved by needles. The pressure via finger or thumb should be deep enough to produce a radiating sensation which is painful but tolerable to the patient. The phrase 'a nice hurt' or 'a good hurt' may explain the apparent

[4] J. A. Lavier, *Points of Chinese Acupuncture*, Health Science Press, England 1974.
[5] Chu-Lien, *Text of Modern Acupuncture*, Public Health Press, Peking, 1956.

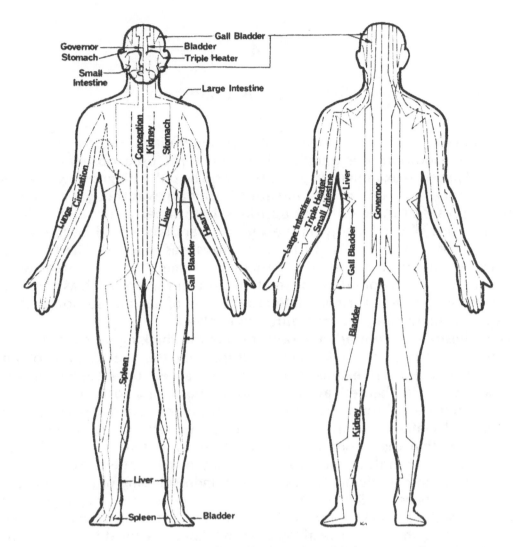

Shows distribution of the twelve bilateral meridians and the two midline meridians
of traditional acupuncture.

contradiction in terms. If the pressure causes the patient to flinch or tense, then it is
too heavy.

It is possible to stimulate several points simultaneously by manual pressure.
When this is being done, it is as well to use variable pressure, easing the depth of
pressure on one point whilst increasing it on the other. Variable pressure is also
useful in treating a single point. Allowing a slow increase and decrease in the
pressure over a ten to twenty-second cycle is a help to the patient and induces
relaxation. Treatment continues until the patient reports an easing of the radiating
discomfort. It is most important not to overdo the degree of stimulation in this form
of acupuncture; use only enough pressure to achieve the 'good hurt', otherwise
bruising and increased discomfort will result.

27

4

When to Use Acupuncture

In traditional acupuncture, treatment was determined largely by the pulse diagnosis. In addition, the traditional acupuncturist used observation, interrogation and physical examination of the patient. The pulse diagnosis was, however, the cornerstone of treatment determination in China. It was thought that by testing the radial pulses at three different positions, both superficially and with deeper pressure, levels of Chi (energy) in the various meridians could be measured. By comparing the various levels of Chi, a diagnosis was reached. The twelve pulse points were evaluated for tension, rate, rhythm, volume, character, intensity, and so on. The findings were considered in relation to other factors, such as age, sex, and temperament, and were further related to the time of day and season of the year. Thus an amazingly complex procedure was evolved.

I would hesitate to contradict the accuracy of this thinking were it not that it has been largely discarded by modern acupuncturists and that the literature of modern China, where the most extensive research is carried on into the validity of acupuncture and its theoretical basis, mentions pulse diagnosis not at all.

I believe it to be in the patient's interest that the practitioner, of whatever school, should use all available means to arrive at a clear understanding of the conditions which exist within the patient. It is certainly feasible that sensitive hands can intuitively sense complex problems in the body of the patient. Such sensitivity, however, must be complemented by a sound understanding of physiological and pathological processes. Since the traditional acupuncturist was steeped in the Taoist philosophy, which dominated all thinking in China, it was natural that medical thinking should evolve along the same lines. We must try to separate the clinical evidence of acupuncture's validity from theories which were evolved to explain the clinical results and which had to conform to a particular philosophical code.

Belief in pulse diagnosis, I suggest, shows a disregard for the knowledge of the structure and function of the human body that exists today. That such knowledge was unknown to Chinese medicine in the past may largely be blamed on the virtually total ban on human dissection in China until modern times. This resulted from the tradition of the veneration of ancestors, which demanded that the body of the deceased should be unmarked by the instruments of dissection or surgery.

Acupuncture should be used when normal diagnosis indicates that it is in the patient's best interest. Pain relief is our present interest and it is in this area of healing that acupuncture offers the most dramatic opportunities for practitioners to help those in their care.

Range of Uses

It can be thought of as a technique, albeit a complex one, and not as a science. A potentially vast range of uses in the treatment of disease and pain is opened up, complementing all methods of physical medicine. We must investigate and utilize all that is valid in the great treasure house of clinical experience that exists in acupuncture literature, but must resist the siren call of its archaic semantics.

In acute traumatic conditions such as whiplash injuries, sprained ankles, and sporting injuries, the use of acupuncture to afford pain relief would be a rational initial approach. In the treatment of early arthritic changes, acupuncture therapy would combine well with physical treatment directed at improving mobility and postural re-education. In more chronic arthritic conditions, acupuncture might afford no more than temporary relief and a more comprehensive approach to the patient would be required.

Treatment by acupuncture is a most useful approach to the so-called 'phantom limb' pains suffered by amputees. It is also helpful in the treatment of causalgia and the neuritis following herpes zoster, and the various facial neuralgias, intercostal neuralgia, and all vague 'nerve' pains, may be all treated symptomatically with it, though underlying causes must be investigated and eliminated, if possible.

Acupuncture is often capable of relieving the colic pains associated with gall stones and kidney stones as well as digestive colic and post-operative distension pain. It is also useful in the treatment of cardiac pain such as angina pectoris. In all such cases it is of course essential to cope with the systemic and organic problems underlying the painful symptoms.

Acupuncture anaesthesia may be employed in surgery and dentistry, though the patient should understand that there will still be sensations of pressure and tension and that the anaesthesia is not total — in fact, deep analgesia is a better description than anaesthesia. It is therefore most important that the patient is completely relaxed, as there is no temporary paralysis of muscles such as occurs in orthodox anaesthesia. The post-operative use of acupuncture is extremely useful in relieving pain and stiffness.

As a first-aid measure in all painful conditions, acupuncture is worthy of trial. All general practitioners, osteopaths, chiropractors, physiotherapists, dentists, nurses and first-aid attendants should have at least a working knowledge of its potential and of its rules. As part of a comprehensive approach to the symptoms of addiction withdrawal, acupuncture is a major step forward.

Some Rules of Acupuncture

To some extent repetition of previously stated procedures is desirable in order to ensure successful treatment and the safety of the patient. It is axiomatic that a correct diagnosis should be arrived at. It is equally important that sound reasons are present for attempting to relieve pain. In the majority of cases this will not be seen as an end in itself, but as part of a comprehensive approach to the resolution of the causes of the patient's problems.

The patient should be co-operative and as relaxed as possible. Elliott[1] states that apprehension is notoriously capable of enhancing the apparent severity of painful conditions, whereas simple mental fortitude can suppress awareness of even massive trauma. This is supported by experienced acupuncturists and those active in the field of acupuncture anaesthesia.[2]

The decision as to whether to use needles, pressure, electrical stimulation or cauterization (moxibustion) must depend on experience. Guidance on this choice as well as the choice of particular points is available in the formulary.

The care of needles is fundamental, as is the degree of asepsis. The points to be treated must be carefully located, and the depth and angle of needle insertion at each point must comply with the advice given in the formulary. If muscular spasm makes insertion difficult, gentle pressure at the periphery of the spasm will induce relaxation. If insertion causes extreme pain, the needle should immediately be withdrawn and another point chosen. The same thing applies if a blood vessel is punctured. The length of stimulation will to some extent be determined by the patient's response, but fifteen to thirty minutes is usually adequate. Removal of the needles must be gentle and slow. The flesh in the area of insertion will grip the needle tightly after manipulation, and this must be allowed to relax so that no further irritation occurs during removal.

In moxibustion treatment, care must be taken not to burn the patient. The raising of a slight blister is permissible in direct cauterization but this is not a technique that should be carried out without experience. The indirect method — heating the handle of the needle — should never be excessively painful for the patient. It is inadvisable to use moxibustion near the sense organs.

In pressure treatment, pain should not be more than is easily tolerable to the patient. The points on the extremities and on the face are rather more sensitive than other points, and more care than usual is therefore required. The patient's attention should be distracted by the physician during insertion of needles in sensitive areas.

If the patient faints during treatment, the needles should immediately be removed and normal action taken to help restore the patient to consciousness.

Extreme care must be taken when needling near the eyes, heart, lungs, liver spleen, spinal cord, or on the thorax or abdomen. Should a needle break after insertion, surgery may be required and delay is inadvisable.

It is inadvisable to treat pregnant women by needle acupuncture anywhere in the sacral area or on the abdomen.

Beginners must pay strict attention to which points are forbidden to needles or moxibustion. Many of the traditionally forbidden points are now used by experienced practitioners, because of the improved flexibility of needles and new techniques of moxibustion, but the newcomer should not attempt to use them until more experienced.

[1]H. C. Elliott, *Textbook of Neuroanatomy* (2nd ed.) Blackwell Scientific Publications, 1969.
[2]*An Outline to Chinese Acupuncture*, Foreign Language Press, Peking, 1975.

5

Auricular Acupuncture

The use of acupuncture points on the external ear in the relief of pain is known as auriculotherapy. This is an ancient method, practised over 2000 years ago, but has been widely used in recent years in China, where active experimentation and clinical use has established many new points. In China, auriculotherapy is used in the treatment of disease in general as well as for pain relief and anaesthesia.

The selection of the points for treatment in auriculotherapy will be assisted by the illustration opposite each formula. Further assistance in localizing the specific point can be obtained in one of the following manners:

1. Press the indicated area with a probe until the most sensitive spot is found. This is the point to treat.
2. Measure the electrical resistance of the skin around the indicated area until the point is found with the lowest resistance to electricity. This is the point to treat.
3. Local physical changes, such as discoloration in the appropriate area if sensitive to pressure, are an indication for treatment at that point.

Treatment of the points on the auricle requires local sterilization, as in general body point treatment. The needle used should be about half an inch long. After penetrating the skin, care must be taken not to pass the needle through the ear.

The patient should feel some discomfort and a sense of local distension. If this is not felt, the needle should be lifted and probed at a slightly different angle until the desired sensation is felt.

Treatment should continue for fifteen to twenty minutes. As in general body acupuncture, the needle should be manipulated by periodical rotating and probing during the treatment. This should be done several times during the period of treatment. To obtain anaesthesia, electro-stimulation of the needle is desirable.

Obviously accuracy is essential in the selection of the point. The degree of success will depend upon this and the subsequent manipulation of the needle.

As a rule, the ear on the side of the painful area should be treated. However, the opposite ear may be treated instead, or both may be treated simultaneously. It may be found that the indicated area is more sensitive to pressure on the ear opposite to the side on which pain is present. In such a case it may be regarded as more appropriate to treat this sensitive point.

Whilst treating the auricular surface it is helpful if the patient is encouraged to gently exercise the painful area.

The majority of points are named for the area upon which they act. Some however, have Chinese names. The appropriate points for treatment in specific conditions will be given in the formulary.

6

Formulary for the Treatment of Pain

In this section the various body areas will be dealt with from the viewpoint of pain relief. Some areas may be further broken down in order to present different formulae for different types of pain, e.g. traumatic injury, neuralgia, arthritis, etc.

Many sections will contain more points than should be used at any one treatment. It is recommended that only one area be treated at any one session. Points should be selected according to the guidelines in Chapter 3. It is quite helpful to combine general body points and auricular points.

Great care has been taken in cross-referencing the points given. Some are a result of my own clinical experience but the majority derive from modern and ancient Chinese sources. Other points are the results of the clinical experience of French, German, American and British workers. There are doubtless other reflex points that are useful in the treatment of pain, but the formulae that follow provide a good starting point in that they are all safe and beneficial if used in the manner previously described.

Remember that digital pressure can be as effective as needling. Needles should be periodically rotated and manipulated during the treatment. In the majority of cases fifteen to twenty minutes of treatment at any one time is adequate. Cauterization often enhances the analgesic effect, especially in rheumatic and arthritic conditions. In acute cases, treatment daily for a week or ten days may be indicated. In chronic conditions, a longer gap between treatments may be allowed, i.e. three days to a week. A course of ten to fifteen treatments over several months followed by a rest period of a month is a useful way of evaluating results in chronically painful conditions.

There is a degree of disagreement regarding the precise location of some points. It has been my practice to define location according to modern Chinese texts. Footnotes concerning such discrepancies will be found in the text.

There is one important point, the location of which causes some confusion. This is Gall Bladder 34, Yang Ling Chüan, and I have given its location as 3 AUM distal to the knee crease in the depression antero-inferior to the small head of the fibula. Most Western authorities give this as postero-inferior to the small head of the fibula.

The point that lies 3 AUM inferior to the knee crease, posterior to the small head of the fibula, is actually a point known as Ling Hou. This is not a meridian point, but is known by the Chinese as a 'strange' point. Its use is indicated in palsy of the leg as well as arthritic knee conditions. It may be that these two points are to some extent interchangeable and it is for this reason that confusion has arisen. Similar discrepancies occur over other points, and the accuracy of some of the descriptions in this book may therefore be queried if compared with certain texts. The only other major area of confusion arises from the variations that occur in the number of units of measurement into which various body areas are divided. The distance from hip to knee crease is often given by Western authorities as 13 AUM, but the more recent Chinese texts give the figure of 19 AUM for the same area. It has been my policy to use the modern Chinese measurement in such cases.

The only major discrepancy between the numbering in this book and recent Chinese publications is the use of the traditional numbering of the bladder meridian rather than the recently altered numbering as published by Chinese authorities. To have altered a major part of the bladder meridian numbers would quite simply have caused too much confusion. It is probably desirable that the Chinese names should be memorized, and repetition of use tends to make this happen without undue effort.

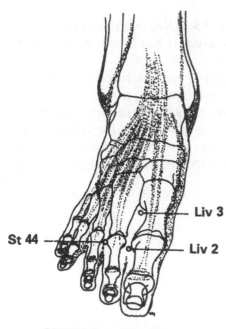

SUPERO — INFERIOR

St 44

Liv 3

Liv 2

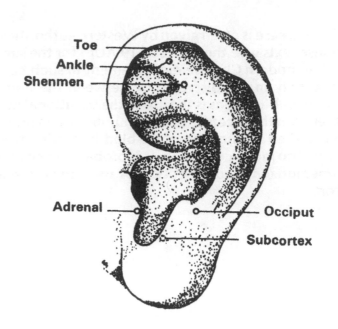

Toe

Ankle

Shenmen

Adrenal

Occiput

Subcortex

LATERAL

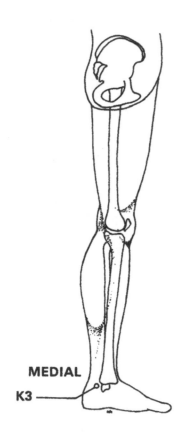

MEDIAL

K3

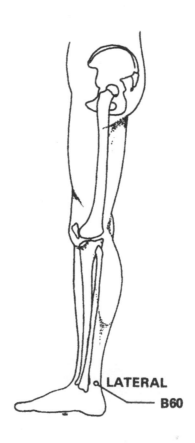

LATERAL

B60

34

FOOT
General Rheumatic or Arthritic Pain

Meridian	Point Ref	Chinese Name	Anatomical Position	Depth of Insertion (inches)	Special Note
LIVER	Liv 2	Hsing Chien	½ AUM proximal to margin of web between 1st and 2nd toes.	¼—½	Slightly oblique insertion required.
KIDNEY	K 3	T'ai Ch'i	Midway between tip of medial malleolus and tendo-calcaneus.	½—1 or ¼—½	Perpendicularly or insert needle towards medial malleolus.
BLADDER	B 60	Kun Lun	Lateral surface of ankle between external malleolus and Achilles tendon. Level with prominence of malleolus.	¾	
LIVER	Liv 3	T'ai Ch'ung	Dorsal surface of foot in angle between 1st and 2nd metatarsals.	¾	Insert needle obliquely upwards.
STOMACH	St 44	Nei T'ing	½ AUM proximal to web margin between 2nd and 3rd toes.	¼—½	Insert at 45° angle inferiorly.

Auricular Points

TOE POINT	Lateral corner of supra-antihelix crus.
ANKLE POINT	Below medial corner of supra-antihelix.
ADRENAL POINT	Lateral border of lower part of tragus.
EAR SHENMEN POINT	Inferior corner of bifurcating point of antihelix.
OCCIPUT POINT	Posterior and superior to lateral aspect of antitragus.
SUBCORTEX POINT	On interior wall of antitragus.

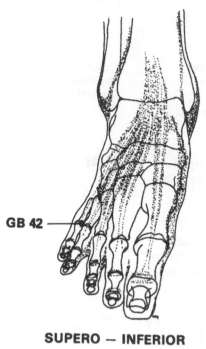

GB 42

SUPERO — INFERIOR

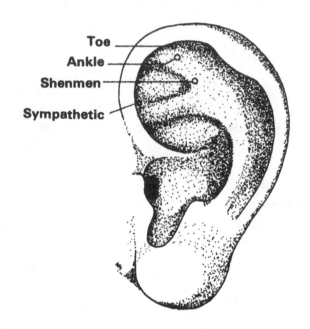

Toe
Ankle
Shenmen
Sympathetic

LATERAL

36

FOOT
Neuralgia (Intermittent Pain).

Meridian	Point Ref	Chinese Name	Anatomical Position	Depth of Insertion (inches)	Special Note
GALL BLADDER	GB 42	Ti Wu Hui	Dorsal surface of foot proximal to and between the metatarsal-phalangeal articulations of the 4th and 5th toes.	¼—½	

Auricular Points

EAR SHENMEN POINT	Inferior corner of bifurcating point of antihelix.
SYMPATHETIC POINT	In deltoid fossa at junction of infra-antihelix crus and medial border of helix.
TOE POINT	Lateral corner of supra-antihelix crus.
ANKLE POINT	Below medial corner of supra-antihelix.

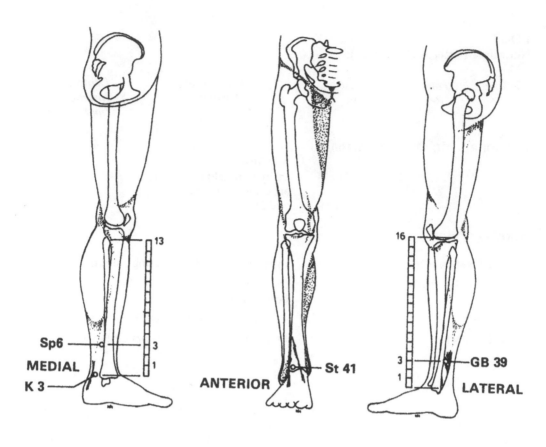

13

Sp6

MEDIAL

K 3

3

1

ANTERIOR

St 41

16

3

1

GB 39

LATERAL

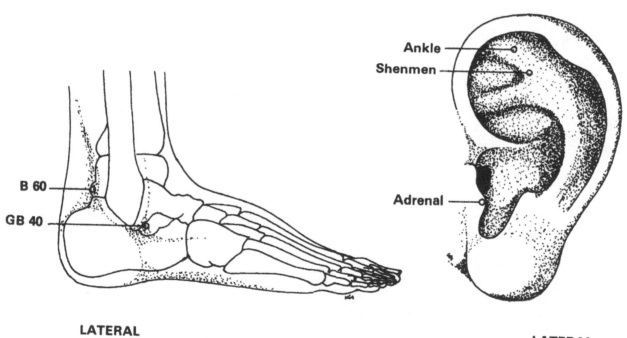

B 60

GB 40

LATERAL

Ankle

Shenmen

Adrenal

LATERAL

ANKLE
Arthritic Pain

Meridian	Point Ref	Chinese Name	Anatomical Position	Depth of Insertion (inches)	Special Note
STOMACH	St 41	Chieh Ch'i	Dorsum of leg. In line with 2nd toe. Between tendons of tibialis anticus and extensor hellucis longus. Level with centre of medial malleolus.	½—1	Indirect cauterization may be helpful.
BLADDER	B 60	Kun Lun	Lateral surface of ankle, between external malleolus and Achilles tendon. Level with prominence of malleolus.	¾	
GALL BLADDER	GB 40	Ch'iu Ch'ü	At the point where anterior and distal margins of lateral malleolus intersect.	½—1	

Auricular Points

ANKLE POINT			Below medial corner of supra-antihelix.		
EAR SHENMEN POINT			Interior corner of bifurcating points of antihelix.		
ADRENAL POINT			Lateral border of lower part of tragus.		

If accompanied by extroversion of the foot, include:

Meridian	Point Ref	Chinese Name	Anatomical Position	Depth of Insertion (inches)	Special Note
KIDNEY	K 3	T' ai Ch'i	Midway between tip of medial malleolus and tendo calcaneus.	½—1 or ¼—½	Perpendicularly or insert towards malleolus.
SPLEEN	Sp 6	San Yin Chiao	3 AUM[1] above tip of internal malleolus, posterior to tibial border.	½—1½	

If accompanied by introversion of the foot, include:

Meridian	Point Ref	Chinese Name	Anatomical Position	Depth of Insertion (inches)	Special Note
GALL BLADDER	GB 39	Hsüan Chung	3 AUM above external malleolus between posterior border of fibula and tendons of peroneus longus and brevis.	½—1	
BLADDER	B 60	Kun Lun	Lateral surface of ankle, between external malleolus and Achilles tendon. Level with prominence of malleolus.	¾	

[1] Note some Western authorities give this as 4 AUM

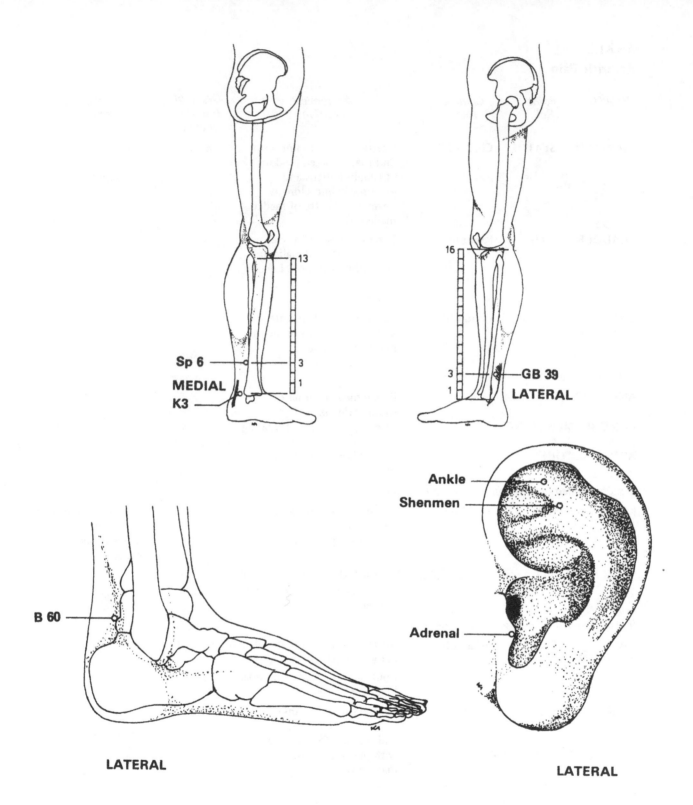

Sp 6

MEDIAL

K3

13

3

1

16

3

1

GB 39

LATERAL

B 60

LATERAL

Ankle

Shenmen

Adrenal

LATERAL

ANKLE
Sprain

Meridian	Point Ref	Chinese Name	Anatomical Position	Depth of Insertion (inches)	Special Note
GALL BLADDER	GB 39	Hsüan Chung	3 AUM above external malleolus.	½—1	Indirect cauterization. Treat Ah Shi points first on the affected limb. If results are not good, treat similar points on the other limb and ask patient to stretch and flex affected joint during treatment.

Ah Shi Points (Local spontaneously sensitive points).

Auricular Points

ANKLE POINT	Below medial corner of supra-antihelix.
EAR SHENMEN POINT	Interior corner of bifurcating point of antihelix.
ADRENAL POINT	Lateral border of lower part of tragus.

If accompanied by extroversion of the foot, include:

Meridian	Point Ref	Chinese Name	Anatomical Position	Depth of Insertion (inches)	Special Note
KIDNEY	K 3	T'ai Ch'i	Midway between tip of medial malleolus and tendo calcaneus.	½—1 or ¼—½	Perpendicularly or insert towards malleolus.
SPLEEN	Sp 6	San Yin Chiao	3 AUM[1] above tip of internal malleolus, posterior to tibial border.	½—1½	

If accompanied by introversion of the foot, include:

Meridian	Point Ref	Chinese Name	Anatomical Position	Depth of Insertion (inches)	Special Note
GALL BLADDER	GB 39	Hsüan Chung	3 AUM above external malleolus between posterior border of fibula and tendons of peroneus longus and brevis.	½—1	
BLADDER	B 60	Kun Lun	Lateral surface of ankle, between external malleolus and Achilles tendon. Level with prominence of malleolus.	¾	

[1] Note some Western authorities give this as 4 AUM

41

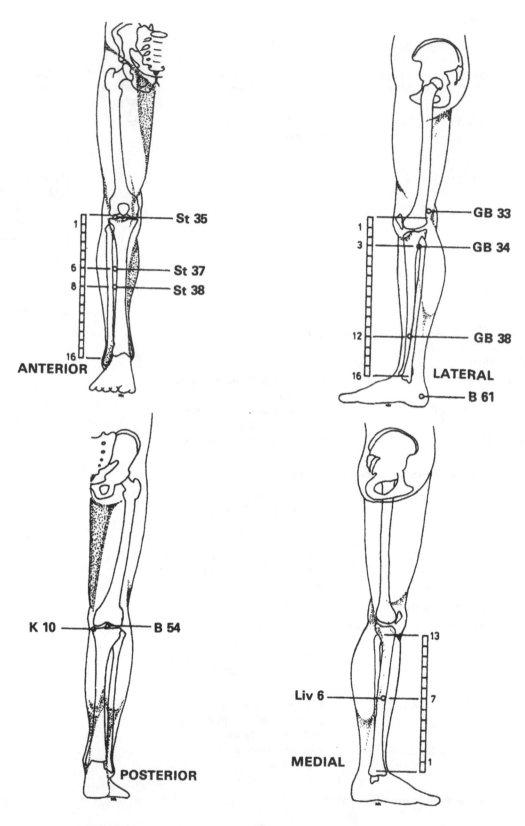

St 35

1

6 St 37
8 St 38

16
ANTERIOR

GB 33

1

3 GB 34

12 GB 38

16 **LATERAL**
B 61

K 10 B 54

POSTERIOR

13

Liv 6 7

MEDIAL 1

42

KNEE
Pain Due to Arthritis of the Knee Joint

Select six to eight points from the following list. Do not choose points on a spontaneously painful site, or on a swelling or tumour. Attempt to encircle the area of pain using points nearest to it. Remember that the contra-lateral joint may be treated to affect the painful joint if the affected area is so swollen as to contra-indicate treatment of it directly.

Meridian	Point Ref	Chinese Name	Anatomical Position	Depth of Insertion (Inches)	Special Note
BLADDER	B 54[1]	Wei Chung	Centre of popliteal crease.	1	Take care regarding artery. Cauterization forbidden.
BLADDER	B 61	Pu Ts'an	Centre of lateral surface of calcaneum.	½	
KIDNEY	K 10	Yin Ku	Medial aspect of popliteal crease when knee flexed. Between semitendinosus muscle and semimembranosus muscle.	1	
GALL BLADDER	GB 33	Yang Kuan	Lateral surface of thigh just proximal to lower head of femur in slight depression.	2	Also useful in sciatic pain. Cauterization forbidden.
GALL BLADDER	GB 34	Yang Ling Ch'üan	Just below head of fibula on lateral surface of leg, 3 AUM below popliteal crease.	2–3	
GALL BLADDER	GB 38	Yang Fu	4 AUM above lateral malleolus in front of fibula.	1	Also for lumbar and general body pain.
LIVER	Liv 6	Chung Tu	Medial aspect of leg, 7 AUM above internal malleolus of the ankle.	½	
STOMACH	St 35	Tu Pi	In depression lateral to patella tendon — just above tibia.	½–1	Slightly slanting insertion medially.
STOMACH	St 37	(Tsu) Shang[2] Lien	Between tibialis anticus and tibia. 6 AUM below knee crease.	2	
STOMACH	St 38	T'iao K'ou	2 AUM below Stomach point 37.	1½	

[1] Note that in recent Chinese literature this point has been renumbered Bladder 40.
[2] Modern Chinese texts name this point Shang Chü Hsü.

continued overleaf

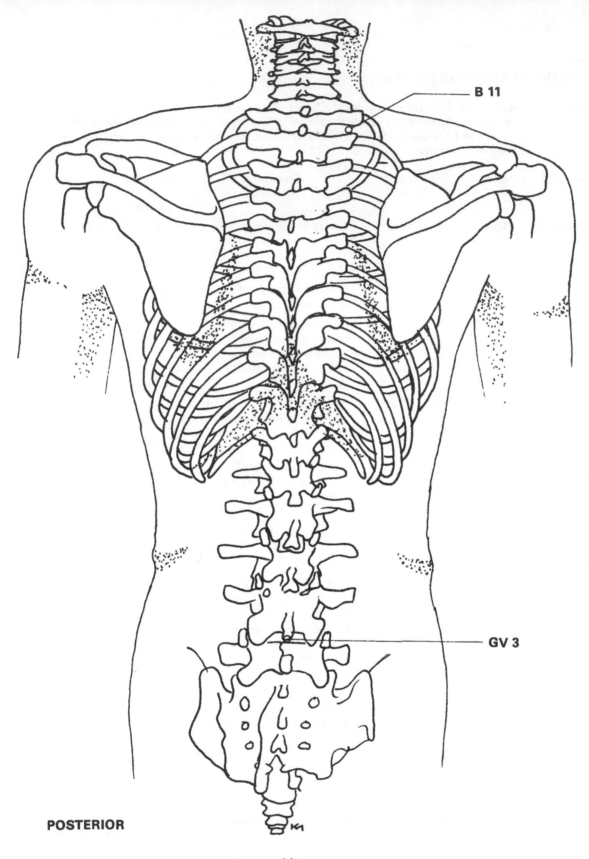

B 11

GV 3

POSTERIOR

44

KNEE
Pain Due to Arthritis of the Knee Joint (contd.)

Meridian	Point Ref	Chinese Name	Anatomical Position	Depth of Insertion (inches)	Special Note
BLADDER	B 11	Ta Chu	Between 1st and 2nd thoracic vertebrae, half way between midline and border of scapula.	½	
GOVERNOR VESSEL	GV 3	Yang Kuan	Between spinous processes of 4th and 5th lumbar vertebrae.	½	Slanting insertion slightly upwards.

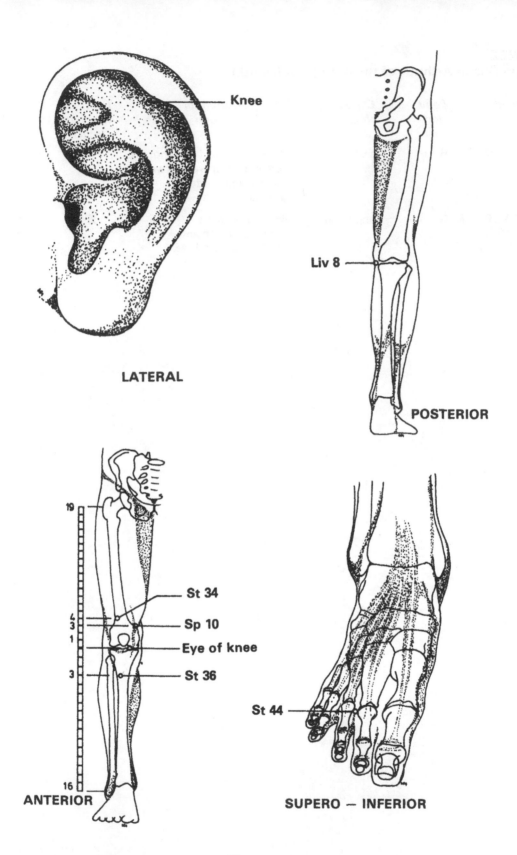

LATERAL

Knee

POSTERIOR

Liv 8

ANTERIOR

St 34
Sp 10
Eye of knee
St 36

19
4
3
1
3
16

SUPERO — INFERIOR

St 44

46

KNEE
General Pain

Meridian	Point Ref	Chinese Name	Anatomical Position	Depth of Insertion (inches)	Special Note
STOMACH	St 34	Liang Ch'iu	4 AUM above knee crease parallel to suprolateral margin of patella.	2	Insert needle at 45° upwards.
STOMACH	St 36	(Tsu) San Li	Anterior surface of leg between tibialis anticus and tibia, 3 AUM below knee joint.	1½—2	Straight insertion.
STOMACH	St 44	Nei T'ing	Dorsal surface of foot between 2nd and 3rd toes just proximal to metatarsal articulation.	¼—½	Insert at 45° angle inferiorly.

Additional Points

To all knee formulae may be added:

1. 'Eye of knee' which lies in depression medial to patella tendon just above tibia (other 'eye of knee' is stomach point 35 (Tu Pi), see previous page). These two points may be used on their own with patient seated, knees flexed.

2. 'Knee joint' point on auricle. At superior crus of antihelix.

3. SPLEEN	Sp 10	Hsüeh Hai	Antero-medial aspect of thigh. 3 AUM above knee, posterior to sartorius muscle.	2	Take care to avoid artery.
LIVER	Liv 8	Ch'ü Ch'üan	At medial end of the knee crease behind lower end of femur.	1	

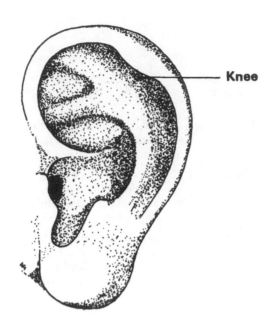

Knee

LATERAL

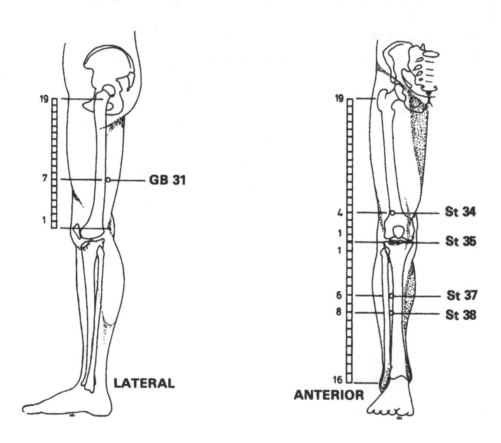

19

7 — **GB 31**

1

LATERAL

19

4 — **St 34**
1
1 — **St 35**

6 — **St 37**
8 — **St 38**

16

ANTERIOR

48

KNEE
Intermittent Pain (Neuralgia)

Meridian	Point Ref	Chinese Name	Anatomical Position	Depth of Insertion (inches)	Special Note
STOMACH	St 34	Liang Ch'iu	2 AUM above patella in line with its lateral margin.	2	Insert needle 45° upwards.
STOMACH	St 35	Tu Pi	In depression lateral to patella tendon — just above tibia.	½—1	Slightly slanting insertion medially.
STOMACH	St 37	(Tsu) Shang[1] Lien	Between tibialis anticus and tibia, 6 AUM below knee crease.	2	
STOMACH	St 38	T'iao K'ou	2 AUM below Stomach 37	1½	
GALL BLADDER	GB 31	Feng Shih	Lateral thigh, 7 AUM above knee crease.	2	

Auricular Point

KNEE POINT			At superior crus of antihelix.		

[1]Modern Chinese texts name this point Shang Chü Hsü.

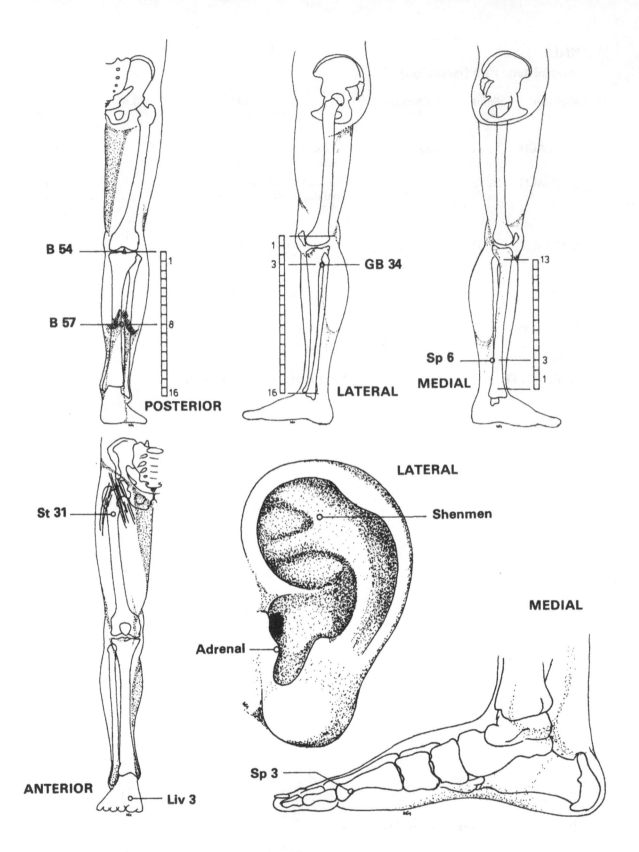

B 54

B 57

1

8

16

POSTERIOR

1

3

GB 34

16

LATERAL

13

Sp 6

3

1

MEDIAL

St 31

ANTERIOR

Liv 3

LATERAL

Shenmen

Adrenal

MEDIAL

Sp 3

50

LOWER LEG
Constant Pain

Meridian	Point Ref	Chinese Name	Anatomical Position	Depth of Insertion (inches)	Special Note
BLADDER	B 57	Ch'eng Shan	8 AUM below knee crease inferior to belly of gastrocnemius.	1—1½	
GALL BLADDER	GB 34	Yang Ling Ch'üan	In depression antero-inferior to small head of fibula.	1—1½	
SPLEEN	Sp 6	San Yin Chiao	3 AUM[1] above tip of internal malleolus posterior to tibial border.	½—1½	Insert slightly inferiorwards.
BLADDER	B 54[2]	Wei Chung	Centre of popliteal crease.	¾—1½	
LIVER	Liv 3	T'ai Ch'ung	Dorsal surface of foot in angle between 1st and 2nd metatarsals.	¾	Insert needle obliquely upwards.
STOMACH	St 31	Pi Kuan	Directly below anterior superior iliac spine, level with lower border of symphasis pubis.	½—1	
SPLEEN	Sp 3	T'ai Pai	Medial aspect of foot posterior and inferior to head of first metatarsal.	¼—½	

Auricular Points

EAR SHENMEN POINT — Inferior corner of bifurcating point of antihelix.

ADRENAL POINT — Lateral border of lower part of tragus.

---

[1] Note some Western authorities give this as 4 AUM.
[2] Note that in recent Chinese literature this point has been renumbered Bladder 40.

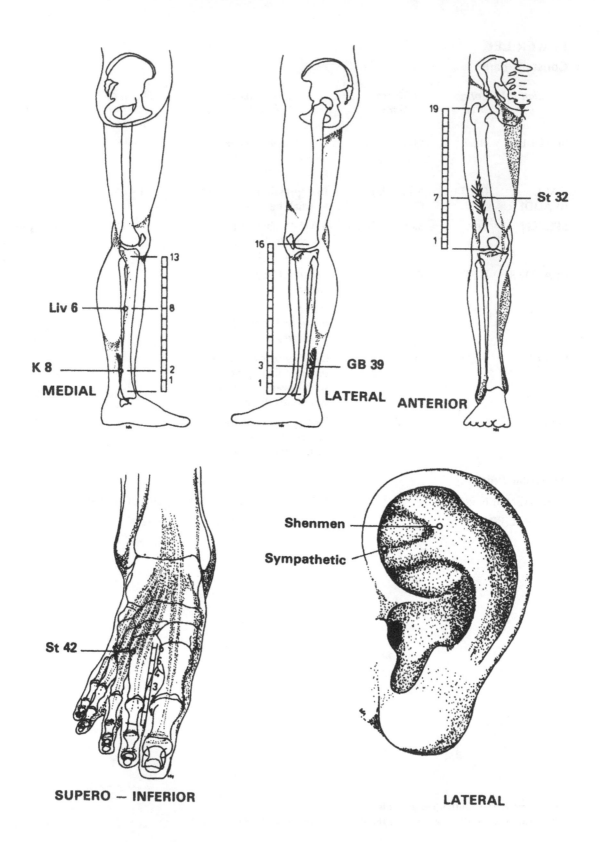

MEDIAL

Liv 6

K 8

13

8

2
1

LATERAL

16

GB 39

3
1

ANTERIOR

19

St 32

7

1

SUPERO — INFERIOR

St 42

LATERAL

Shenmen

Sympathetic

LOWER LEG
Neuralgia (Intermittent Pain)

Meridian	Point Ref	Chinese Name	Anatomical Position	Depth of Insertion (inches)	Special Note
KIDNEY	K 8	Chiao Hsin	Internal surface of leg 2 AUM[1] above malleolus between tibia and flexor digitorum longus.	½—1	
GALL BLADDER	GB 39	Hsüan Chung	3 AUM above external malleolus between posterior border of fibula and tendons of peroneus longus and brevis.	½—1	
LIVER	Liv 6	Chung Tu	8 AUM[2] above medial malleolus, posterior to edge of tibia.	½—1½	Perpendicular or oblique insertion.
STOMACH	St 32	Fu Tu	Located on anterior surface of thigh 7 AUM above popliteal crease; between rectus femoris and vastus lateralis.	1—1½	Insert along lateral border of femur.
STOMACH	St 42	Ch'ung Yang	Highest point of dorsum of foot 5½ AUM proximal to web margin between 2nd and 3rd toes.	½	Take care to avoid artery.

Auricular Points

EAR SHENMEN POINT	Inferior corner of bifurcating point of antihelix.
SYMPATHETIC NERVE POINT	In deltoid fossa at junction of infra-antihelix crus and medial border of helix.

---

[1] Some Western authorities give this as 3 AUM.

[2] Note that some Western authorities give this as 7 AUM above internal malleolus.

53

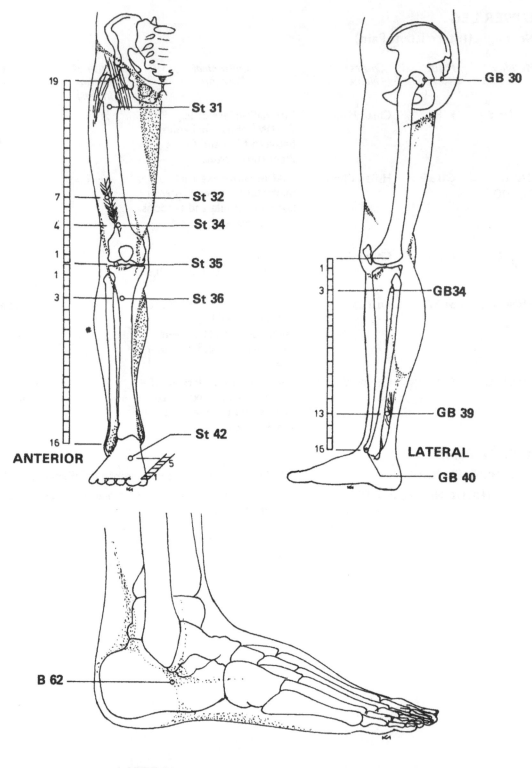

ANTERIOR

19 — St 31
7 — St 32
4 — St 34
1 — St 35
1
3 — St 36
16 — St 42
5

LATERAL

GB 30
1
3 — GB34
13 — GB 39
16 — GB 40

B 62

LATERAL

LEG
General Pain

Choose from the following:

Meridian	Point Ref	Chinese Name	Anatomical Position	Depth of Insertion (inches)	Special Note
BLADDER	B 62	Shen Mei	Directly below lateral malleolus in a depression.	¼—½	
GALL BLADDER	GB 30	Huan T'iao	Patient side lying thigh flexed, ⅓ of distance from greater trochanter to the sacral hiatus.	1½—3	
	GB 34	Yang Ling Chüan	In depression antero-inferior to small head of fibula.	1—1½	
	GB 39	Hsüan Chung	3 AUM above lateral malleolus, between border of fibula and tendons of peroneus longus and brevis.	½—1	
	GB 40	Ch'iu Ch'ü	At the point where anterior and distal margins of the lateral malleolus intersect.	½—1	
STOMACH	St 31	Pi Kuan	Directly below anterior-superior iliac spine, level with lower border of symphasis pubis.	½—1	
	St 32	Fu Tu	Anterior surface of thigh 7 AUM above popliteal crease, between rectus femoris and vastus lateralis.	1—1½	
	St 34	Liang Ch'iu	4 AUM above knee crease parallel to supro-lateral margin of patella.	1	
	St 35	Tu Pi	In depression lateral to patella in line with its lateral margin.	½—1	Insert obliquely and medially.
	St 36	(Tsu) San Li	3 AUM below tupi, one finger's width lateral to crest of tibia.	1—1½	
	St 42	Ch'ung Yang	Highest point of dorsum of foot 5½ AUM proximal to web margin between 2nd and 3rd toes.	½	Take care to avoid artery.

continued overleaf

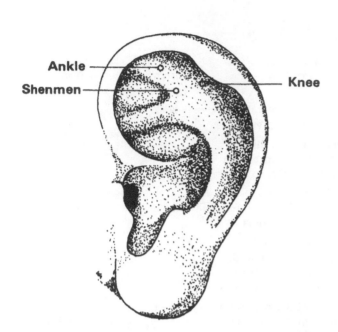

Ankle
Shenmen
Knee

LATERAL

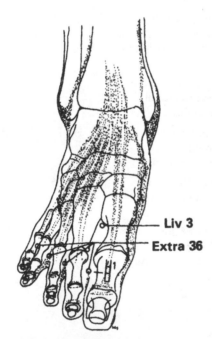

Liv 3
Extra 36

SUPERO — INFERIOR

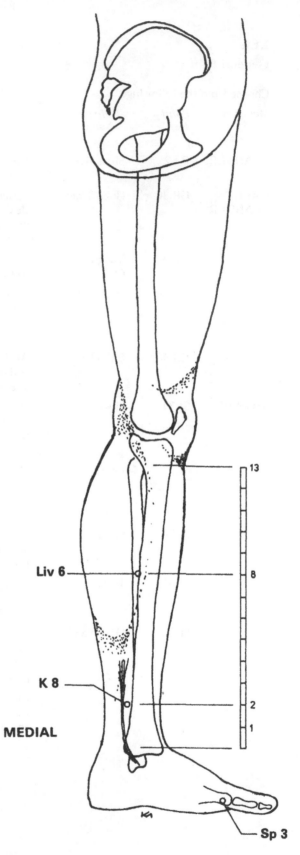

Liv 6
K 8
Sp 3

13
8
2
1

MEDIAL

56

LEG
General Pain (contd.)

Meridian	Point Ref	Chinese Name	Anatomical Position	Depth of Insertion (inches)	Special Note
LIVER	Liv 3	T'ai Ch'ung	Dorsal surface of foot in angle between 1st and 2nd metatarsals.	¾	Insert needle obliquely upwards.
	Liv 6	Chung Tu	Medial aspect of leg 8 AUM above medial malleolus, posterior to edge of tibia.	½–1½	Perpendicular or oblique insertion.
SPLEEN	Sp 3	T'ai Pai	Medial aspect of foot posterior and inferior to head of the 1st metatarsal.	¼–½	
KIDNEY	K 8	Chiao Hsin	Internal Surface of leg 2 AUM[1] above malleolus between tibia and flexor digitorum longus.	½–1	
EXTRA 36		Ba Feng	On the dorsum of the foot ½ AUM proximal to the web of toes (total of 8 points).	½	Insert obliquely upwards.

Auricular Points

ANKLE POINT		Below medial corner of supra-antihelix
EAR SHENMEN POINT		Inferior corner of bifurcating point of antihelix.
KNEE POINT		At superior crus of antihelix.

[1] Some Western authorities give this as 3 AUM.

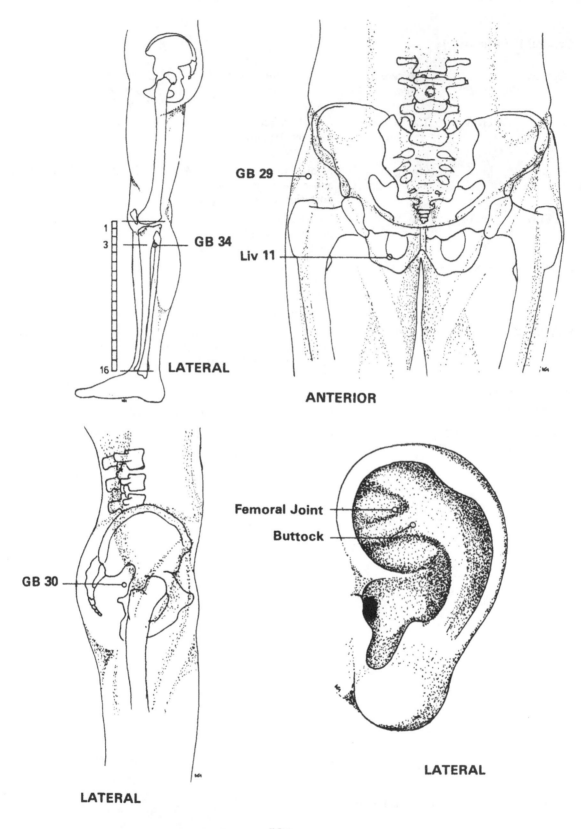

GB 34

GB 29

Liv 11

LATERAL

ANTERIOR

GB 30

LATERAL

Femoral Joint

Buttock

LATERAL

58

HIP
Arthritic Pain and General Pain

Meridian	Point Ref	Chinese Name	Anatomical Position	Depth of Insertion (inches)	Special Note
GALL BLADDER	GB 30	Huan T'iao	Patient side lying, thigh flexed, $\frac{1}{3}$ of the distance between greater trochanter and sacral hiatus.	2—3	Cauterization useful.
GALL BLADDER	GB 34	Yang Ling Ch'üan	In the depression antero-inferior to small head of fibula.	1—1½	
GALL BLADDER	GB 29	Chü Liao	Midway between anterior superior iliac spine and highest point of greater trochanter of femur.	1—2	
LIVER	Liv 11	Yin Lien	On the flexure of the groin lateral to femoral artery.	1—1½	Insert needle slightly laterally.

Auricular Points

BUTTOCK POINT   Midpoint, lateral aspect infra-antihelix crus.

FEMORAL JOINT POINT   In lateral third of lower border of deltoid fossa.

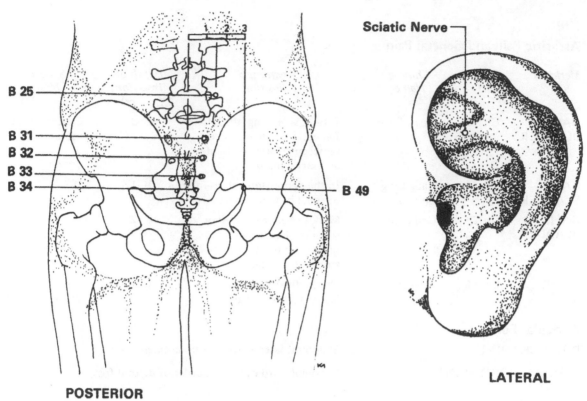

B 25

B 31
B 32
B 33
B 34

B 49

Sciatic Nerve

POSTERIOR

LATERAL

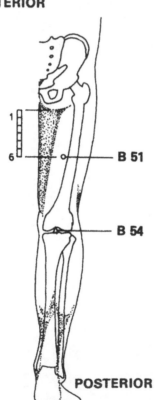

B 51

B 54

POSTERIOR

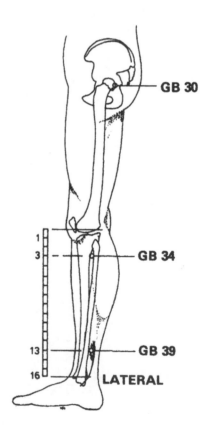

GB 30

GB 34

GB 39

LATERAL

SCIATIC PAIN

Meridian	Point Ref	Chinese Name	Anatomical Position	Depth of Insertion (inches)	Special Note
BLADDER	B 49[1]	Chih Pien	3 AUM lateral to midline on level of the 4th sacral foramen.	1½—2	
BLADDER	B 25	Ta Ch'ang Yü	1½ AUM lateral to lower border of spinous process of 4th lumbar vertebra.	1—1½	
BLADDER	B 31	Shang Liao	In the 1st sacral foramen.	1¼	
BLADDER	B 32	Tz'ǔ Liao	in the 2nd sacral foramen.	1¼	
BLADDER	B 33	Chung Liao	In the 3rd sacral foramen.	1¼	
BLADDER	B 34	Hsia Liao	In the 4th sacral foramen.	1¼	
BLADDER	B 51[2]	Yin Men	6 AUM below gluteal fold on median line of leg.	1—2	Sensation should radiate to foot.
BLADDER	B 54[3]	Wei Chung	Exact centre of politeal crease.	¾—1½	Allow to bleed if possible. Cauterization forbidden.
GALL BLADDER	GB 30	Huan T'iao	Patient side lying, thigh flexed ⅓ of distance between greater trochanter and sacral hiatus.	2—3	
GALL BLADDER	GB 34	Yang Ling Ch'üan	In depression antero-inferior to small head of fibula.	1—1½	
GALL BLADDER	GB 39	Hsüan Chung	3 AUM above external malleolus between posterior border of fibula and tendons of peroneus longus and brevis.	½—1	

Auricular Point

SCIATIC NERVE POINT			On midpoint of medial aspect of infra-antihelix crus.		

[1] In new texts the Chinese number this Bladder 54.
[2] In new texts the Chinese number this Bladder 37.
[3] Note that in recent Chinese literature this point has been renumbered Bladder 40.

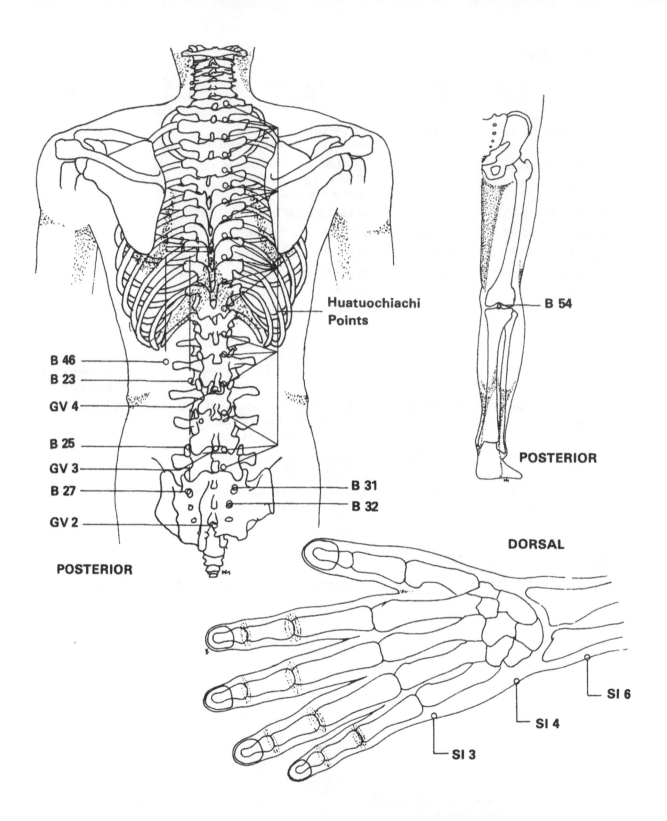

Huatuochiachi
Points

B 46
B 23
GV 4

B 25
GV 3
B 27
GV 2

B 31
B 32

POSTERIOR

B 54

POSTERIOR

DORSAL

SI 6
SI 4
SI 3

LUMBAR PAIN

Meridian	Point Ref	Chinese Name	Anatomical Position	Depth of Insertion (inches)	Special Note
BLADDER	B 23	Shen Yü	1½ AUM lateral to inferior border of spinous process of 2nd lumbar vertebra.[1]	1–1½	
BLADDER	B 46	Huang Men	3 AUM lateral to inferior border of 1st lumbar vertebra.	¾	
BLADDER	B 54[2]	Wei Chung	Exact centre of popliteal crease.	¾–1½	Cauterization forbidden.
SMALL INTESTINE	SI 4	Wan Ku	Ulna border of palm in a depression, proximal to 5th metacarpal.	¼	
SMALL INTESTINE	SI 6	Yang Lao	1 AUM above styloid process of ulna on posterior surface of forearm.	1	

For rheumatic pain, add:

Meridian	Point Ref	Chinese Name	Anatomical Position	Depth of Insertion (inches)	Special Note
BLADDER	B 25	Ta Ch'ang Yü	1½ AUM lateral to inferior border of spinous process of 4th lumbar vertebra.	1	
BLADDER	B 27	Hsiao Ch'ang Yü	1½ AUM lateral to midline at level of 1st sacral foramen.	¾	
BLADDER	B 31	Shang Liao	In 1st sacral foramen.	1	
BLADDER	B 32	Tz'ŭ Liao	In 2nd sacral foramen.	1	
GOVERNOR VESSEL	GV 2	Yao Yü	Sacro-coccygeal articulation.	¾	Angle needle upwards.
GOVERNOR VESSEL	GV 3	Yang Kuan	Between 4th and 5th lumbar vertebrae.	1¼	Angle needle slightly upwards.
GOVERNOR VESSEL	GV 4	Ming Men	Between 2nd and 3rd lumbar vertebra.	1¼	

For lumbar sprain, add:

Meridian	Point Ref	Chinese Name	Anatomical Position	Depth of Insertion (inches)	Special Note
SMALL INTESTINE	SI 3	Hou Ch'i	On the transverse crease proximal to 5th metacarpophalangeal joint.	¼	

[1] In very acute cases distal points should be used, in addition to local points. Electro-acupuncture as well as cauterization may be useful.

[2] Note that in recent Chinese literature this point has been renumbered Bladder 40.

continued overleaf

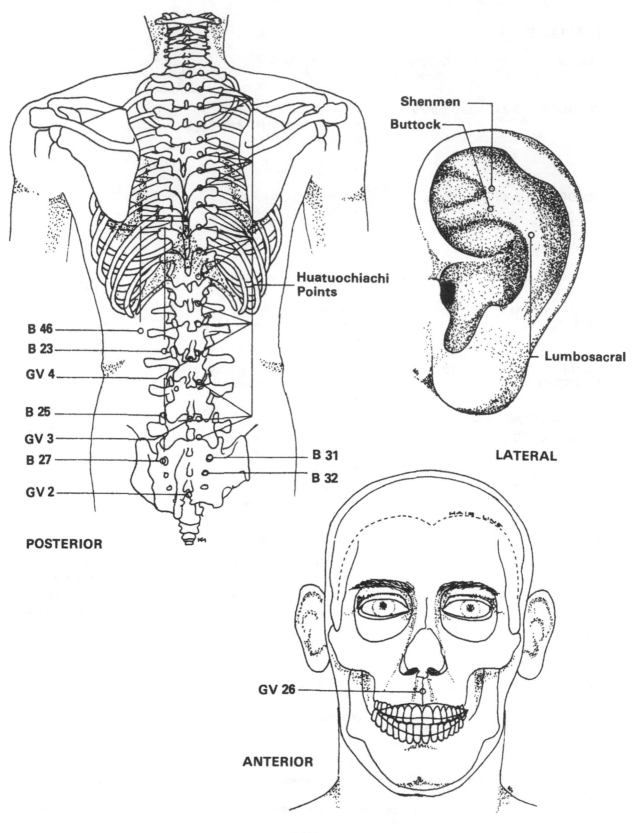

Shenmen

Buttock

Huatuochiachi
Points

B 46

B 23

GV 4

B 25

GV 3

B 27

GV 2

B 31

B 32

Lumbosacral

LATERAL

POSTERIOR

GV 26

ANTERIOR

64

LUMBAR PAIN (contd.)

Meridian	Point Ref	Chinese Name	Anatomical Position	Depth of Insertion (inches)	Special Note
GOVERNOR VESSEL	GV 26	Shui Kou	Median line of face, below nose. Centre of philtrum.	¼	

Select additional points from:

HUATUOCHIACHI POINTS — On both sides spinal column, ½ AUM lateral to midline on level of superior aspect of transverse processes. Select according to sensitivity. Insert needle 1½" slightly obliquely towards spinal column in lumbar area. 1" in thoracic area.

Auricular Points

LUMBOSACRAL POINT — On the medial border of antihelix.

BUTTOCK POINT — Midpoint of lateral aspect of infra-antihelix crus.

EAR SHENMEN POINT — Inferior corner of bifurcating point of antihelix.

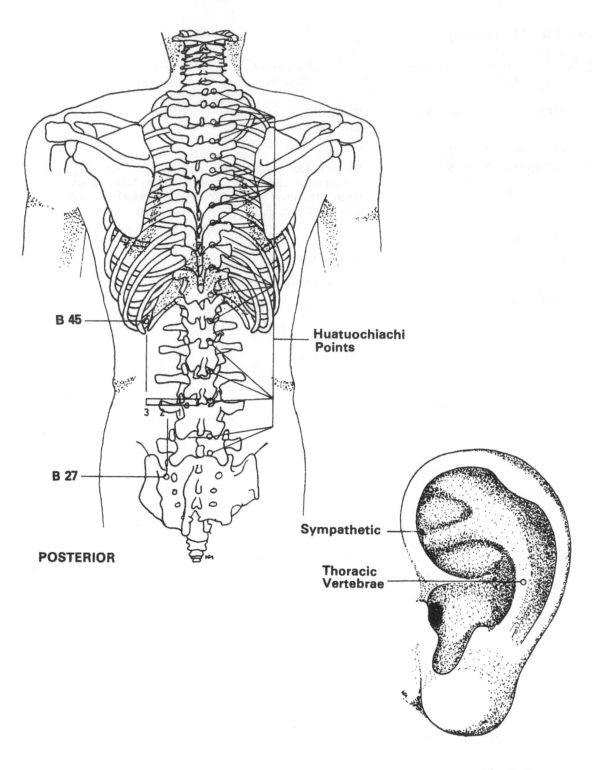

B 45

Huatuochiachi
Points

B 27

POSTERIOR

Sympathetic

Thoracic
Vertebrae

LATERAL

66

DORSAL SPINE PAIN

Meridian	Point Ref	Chinese Name	Anatomical Position	Depth of Insertion (inches)	Special Note
BLADDER	B 27	Hsiao Ch'ang Yü	1½ AUM lateral to median line. Level of 1st sacral foramen.	1	
BLADDER	B 45	Wei Ts'ang	3 AUM lateral to spine. Level of intervertebral depression between 12th dorsal vertebra and 1st lumbar.	1	
HUATUOCHIACHI POINTS			On both sides of the spinal column. ½ AUM lateral to midline on level of superior aspect of transverse processes. Select according to sensitivity. Insert needle 1″ slightly obliquely towards spinal column.		

Auricular Points

THORACIC VERTEBRA POINT	Centre of medial border of antihelix.
SYMPATHETIC NERVE POINT	In deltoid fossa at junction of infra-antihelix crus and medial border of helix.

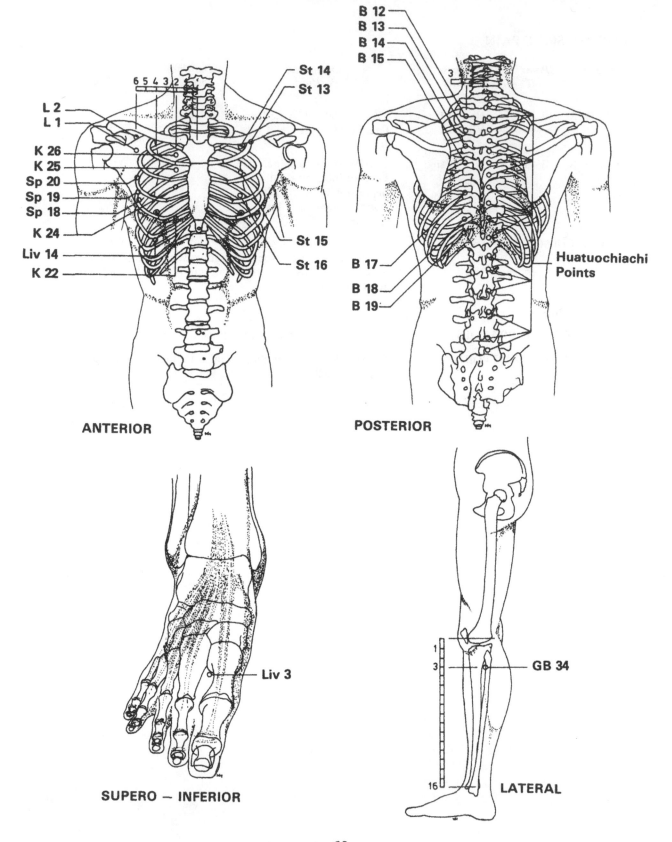

ANTERIOR

POSTERIOR

SUPERO – INFERIOR

LATERAL

INTERCOSTAL NEURALGIA

Select 6 or 7 of the following points at each treatment:

Meridian	Point Ref	Chinese Name	Anatomical Position	Depth of Insertion (inches)	Special Note
BLADDER	B 12	Fêng Men	1½ AUM lateral to lower border of spinous process of 2nd thoracic vertebra.	$\frac{1}{3}$	
BLADDER	B 13	Fei Yü	1½ AUM lateral to lower border of spinous process of 3rd thoracic vertebra.	$\frac{1}{3}$	
BLADDER	B 14	Chuëh Yin Yü	1½ AUM lateral to lower border of spinous process of 4th thoracic vertebra.	$\frac{1}{3}$	
BLADDER	B 15	Hsin Yü	1½ AUM lateral to lower border of spinous process of 5th thoracic vertebra.	$\frac{1}{3}$	
BLADDER	B 17	Ko Yü	1½ AUM lateral to lower border of spinous process of 7th thoracic vertebra.	$\frac{1}{3}$	
BLADDER	B 18	Kan Yü	1½ AUM lateral to lower border of spinous process of 9th thoracic vertebra.	$\frac{1}{3}$	
BLADDER	B 19	Tan Yü	1½ AUM lateral to lower border of spinous process of 10th thoracic vertebra.	$\frac{1}{3}$	
KIDNEY	K 22	Pu Lang	2 AUM lateral to midline in 5th intercostal space.	½	
KIDNEY	K 24	Ling Ch'ü	2 AUM lateral to midline in 3rd intercostal space.	½	
KIDNEY	K 25	Shen Ts'ang	2 AUM lateral to midline in 2nd intercostal space.	½	
KIDNEY	K 26	Huo Chung	2 AUM lateral to midline in 1st intercostal space.	½	
LIVER	Liv 14	Ch'i Men	On mammillary line in the intercostal space of 6th and 7th ribs.	¾	
LIVER	Liv 3	T'ai Ch'ung	Dorsal surface of foot 2 AUM proximal to web between 1st and 2nd toes.	¾	
GALL BLADDER	GB 34	Yang Ling Ch'üan	In depression antero-inferior to small head of fibula.	1	
STOMACH	St 13	Ch'i Hu	In depression inferior to midpoint of clavicle.	½	
STOMACH	St 14	K'u Fang	1st intercostal space upon mammillary line.	½	

continued overleaf

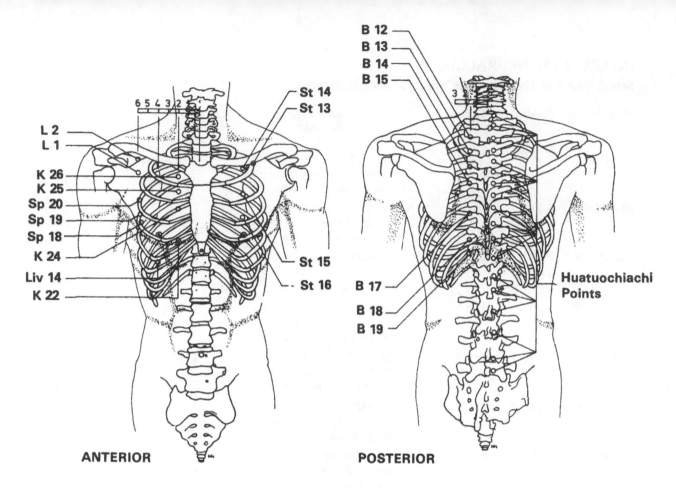

St 14
St 13

L 2
L 1

K 26
K 25
Sp 20
Sp 19
Sp 18
K 24
Liv 14
K 22

6 5 4 3 2

St 15
St 16

ANTERIOR

B 12
B 13
B 14
B 15

3 2

B 17
B 18
B 19

Huatuochiachi
Points

POSTERIOR

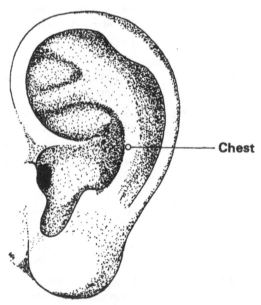

Chest

LATERAL

INTERCOSTAL NEURALGIA
Select 6 or 7 of the following points at each treatment: (contd.)

Meridian	Point Ref	Chinese Name	Anatomical Position	Depth of Insertion (inches)	Special Note
STOMACH	St 15	Wu I	Above nipple in 2nd intercostal space.	½	
STOMACH	St 16	Ying Ch'uang	Above nipple in 3rd intercostal space.	½	
LUNG	L 1	Chung Fu	On lateral aspect of chest, 6 AUM from midline in 1st intercostal space.	½	Lateral insertion.
LUNG	L 2	Yün Men	Below the clavicle, 6 AUM lateral to midline.	¾	
SPLEEN	Sp 18	T'ien Ch'i	In 4th intercostal space, 6 AUM lateral to midline.	½	
SPLEEN	Sp 19	Hsiung Hsiang	In 3rd intercostal space, 6 AUM lateral to midline.	½	
SPLEEN	Sp 20	Cho Jung	In 2nd intercostal space, 6 AUM lateral to midline.	½	
HUATUOCHIACHI POINTS			On both sides of spinal column, ½ AUM lateral to midline on level of superior aspect of transverse processes. Select according to sensitivity. Insert 1" obliquely towards spinal column.		

Auricular Point

CHEST POINT	Antihelix on level of supra-tragic notch.

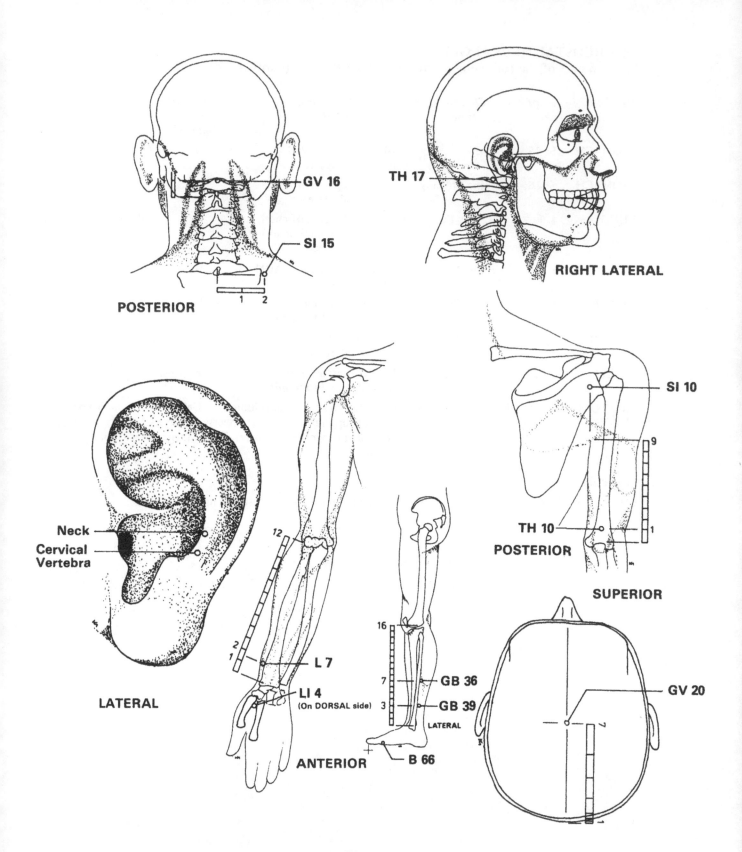

POSTERIOR

GV 16

SI 15

RIGHT LATERAL

TH 17

Neck

Cervical
Vertebra

LATERAL

L 7

LI 4
(On DORSAL side)

ANTERIOR

SI 10

TH 10

POSTERIOR

SUPERIOR

GB 36

GB 39

LATERAL

B 66

GV 20

72

NECK

General Pain

Choose from the following points (not more than 6 at any one time):

Meridian	Point Ref	Chinese Name	Anatomical Position	Depth of Insertion (inches)	Special Note
GOVERNOR VESSEL	GV 20	Pai Hui	On midline of skull 7 AUM proximal to posterior hairline.	¼	Horizontally inferiorly.
GOVERNOR VESSEL	GV 16	Fēng Fu	Inferior to occipital protuberance 1 AUM above hairline in a depression.	½	
LUNG	L 7	Lieh Ch'üeh	1½ AUM proximal to transverse wrist crease above styloid process of radius.	½	Needle insertion obliquely upwards.
SMALL INTESTINE	SI 10	Nao Yü	With arm at side, directly above posterior axilliary fold. In depression below spine of scapula.	1	
SMALL INTESTINE	SI 15	Chien Chung Yü	2 AUM lateral to inferior aspect of spinous process of 7th cervical vertebra.	¾	

For the lower neck add:

Meridian	Point Ref	Chinese Name	Anatomical Position	Depth of Insertion (inches)	Special Note
BLADDER	B 66	(Yang) Tung Ku	In a depression antero-lateral to 5th metatarso-phalangeal joint.	¼	
GALL BLADDER	GB 36	Wai Ch'iu	7 AUM above lateral malleolus, posterior to fibula.	1	
GALL BLADDER	GB 39	Hsüan Chung	3 AUM above lateral malleolus, posterior to fibula.	1	
TRIPLE HEATER	TH 10	T'ien Ching	1 AUM posterior and superior to olecrenon. In a depression formed on flexing of elbow.	¾	
TRIPLE HEATER	TH 17	I Fêng	Between mastoid process and mandible, posterior to ear-lobe.	1	Slightly anteriorly and superiorly.
LARGE INTESTINE	LI 4	Ho Ku	Dorsal surface of hand in angle between 1st 2 metacarpals.	1	

Auricular Points

CERVICAL VERTEBRA POINT	Lower medial aspect of antihelix.
NECK POINT	At junction of antihelix and antitragus.

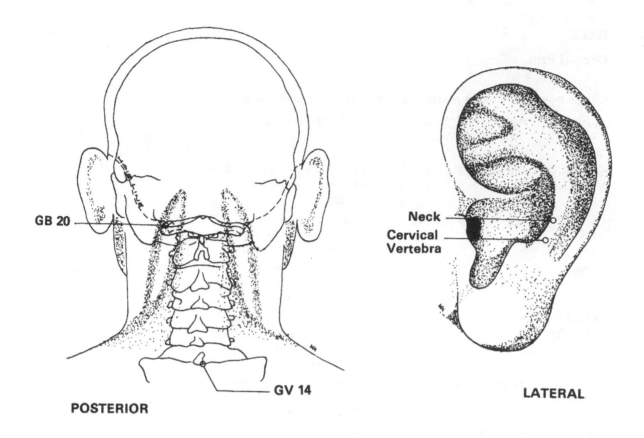

GB 20

GV 14

POSTERIOR

Neck

Cervical
Vertebra

LATERAL

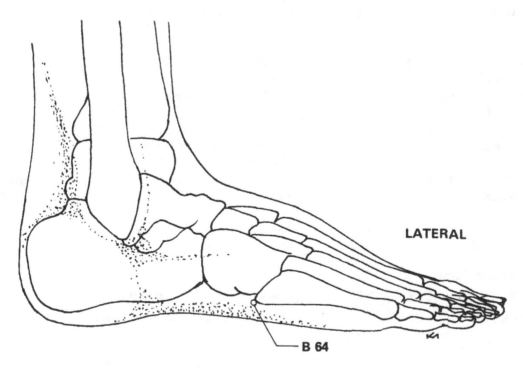

LATERAL

B 64

74

NECK
Whiplash Injury

Meridian	Point Ref	Chinese Name	Anatomical Position	Depth of Insertion (inches)	Special Note
GALL BLADDER	GB 20	Fêng Ch'ih	Between depression inferior to occipital protuberance and mastoid bone.	1	Needle towards orbit on opposite side. No deeper than indicated.
GOVERNOR VESSEL	GV 14	Ta Ch'ui	Between 7th cervical vertebra and 1st thoracic vertebra.	1	No deeper than indicated.
BLADDER	B 64	Ching Ku	External surface of foot, below tuberosity of 5th metatarsal.	½	

Auricular Points

CERVICAL VERTEBRA POINT	Lower medial aspect of antihelix.
NECK POINT	At junction of antihelix and antitragus.

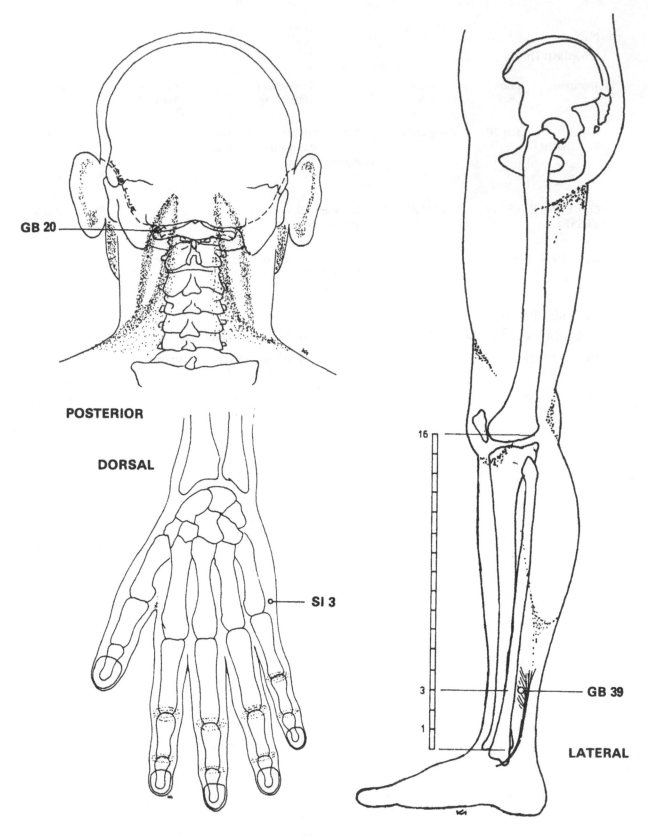

GB 20

POSTERIOR

DORSAL

SI 3

16

3

GB 39

1

LATERAL

76

NECK
Torticollis

Use Ah Shi (local spontaneously tender) points on neck and shoulders.

Add:

Meridian	Point Ref	Chinese Name	Anatomical Position	Depth of Insertion (inches)	Special Note
GALL BLADDER	GB 20	Fêng Ch'ih	Between depression inferior to occipital protuberance and the mastoid bone.	1	Needle towards orbit on opposite side. No deeper than indicated.
GALL BLADDER	GB 39	Hsüan Chung	3 AUM above lateral malleolus, between fibula and tendon of peroneus longus.	¾	
SMALL INTESTINE	SI 3	Hou Ch'i	Medial aspect transverse palmer crease, proximal to 5th metacarpo-phalangeal joint (with hand making a fist).	¾	

Auricular Points

CERVICAL VERTEBRA POINT — Lower medial aspect of antihelix.

NECK POINT — At junction of antihelix and antitragus.

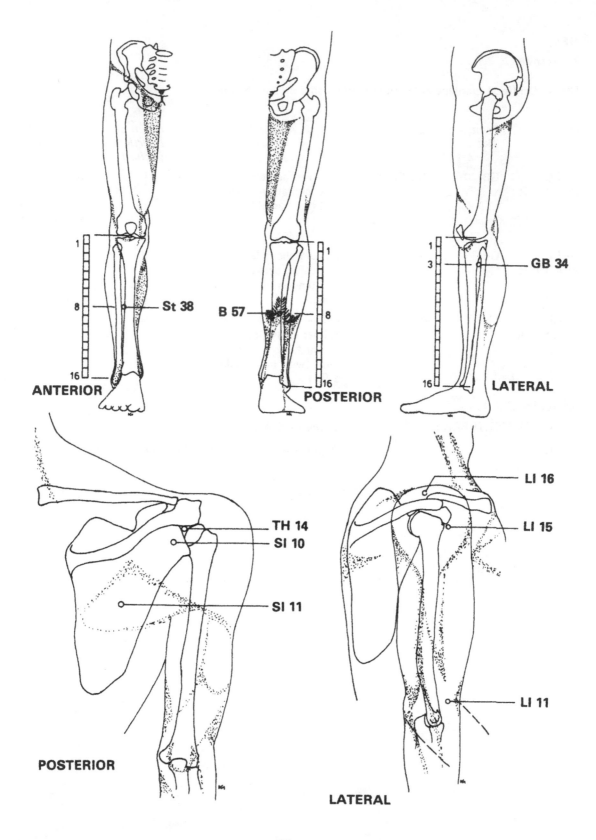

ANTERIOR

St 38

1
8
16

POSTERIOR

B 57

1
8
16

LATERAL

GB 34

1
3
16

POSTERIOR

TH 14
SI 10
SI 11

LATERAL

LI 16
LI 15
LI 11

SHOULDER PAIN

Combine the following two points: direct the needle from Stomach 38 towards Bladder 57; or needles may be inserted into both.

Meridian	Point Ref	Chinese Name	Anatomical Position	Depth of Insertion (inches)	Special Note
STOMACH	St 38	T'iao Kou	8 AUM below knee crease between tibialis anticus and tibia.	1½	
BLADDER	B 57	Ch'eng Shan	8 AUM below knee crease inferior to belly of gastrocnemius.	1¼	

Also useful in general shoulder pain are:

Meridian	Point Ref	Chinese Name	Anatomical Position	Depth of Insertion (inches)	Special Note
LARGE INTESTINE	LI 15	Chien Yü	Anterio-inferior aspect of the acromion. In depression when arm raised.	¾—1	Perpendicularly, unless arm abducted, in which case obliquely downwards.
SMALL INTESTINE	SI 10	Nao Yü	With arm at side, directly above posterior axillary fold. In depression below spine of scapula.	1	
LARGE INTESTINE	LI 11	Ch'ü Ch'ih	At external aspect of elbow crease with elbow flexed. Between lateral epicondyle and edge of elbow fold.	1¼	
GALL BLADDER	GB 34	Yang Ling Ch'üan	In depression antero-inferior to small head of fibula.	1¼	

For bursitis, add:

Meridian	Point Ref	Chinese Name	Anatomical Position	Depth of Insertion (inches)	Special Note
SMALL INTESTINE	SI 11	T'ien Tsung	Centre of infrascapular fossa. Level with 4th thoracic spinous process.	¾	

For chronic degenerative changes, add:

Meridian	Point Ref	Chinese Name	Anatomical Position	Depth of Insertion (inches)	Special Note
LARGE INTESTINE	LI 16	Chü Ku	In depression between acromial end of clavicle and superior aspect of spine of scapula.	1	

For pain on lateral aspect, add:

Meridian	Point Ref	Chinese Name	Anatomical Position	Depth of Insertion (inches)	Special Note
TRIPLE HEATER	TH 14	Chien Liao	Postero-inferior aspect of the acromion process at same level as Large Intestine 15.	1¼	Direct needle between acromion and greater tubercle; arm abducted to horizontal.

continued overleaf

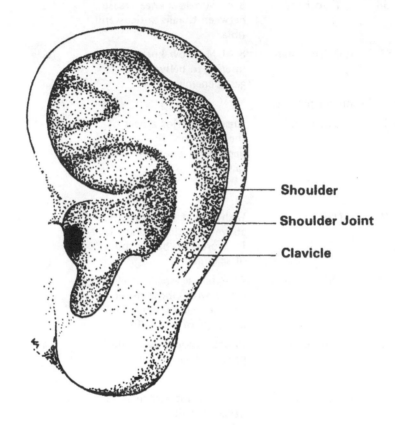

Shoulder

Shoulder Joint

Clavicle

LATERAL

80

SHOULDER PAIN (contd.)

For inflamed biceps tendon, add:

Ah Shi (local spontaneously tender) points.
As with other conditions, distant points may be used, during which time the joint should be moved gently; e.g. Gall Bladder 34 or Stomach 38 (see above).

Auricular Points

SHOULDER POINT	In scapha, level with supra-tragic notch.
SHOULDER JOINT POINT	Between shoulder point and clavicle point.
CLAVICLE POINT	In scapha at level of junction of antihelix and antitragus.

All points should be strongly stimulated. Electro-acupuncture and moxibustion is useful. Choose 5 or 6 points at any one treatment.

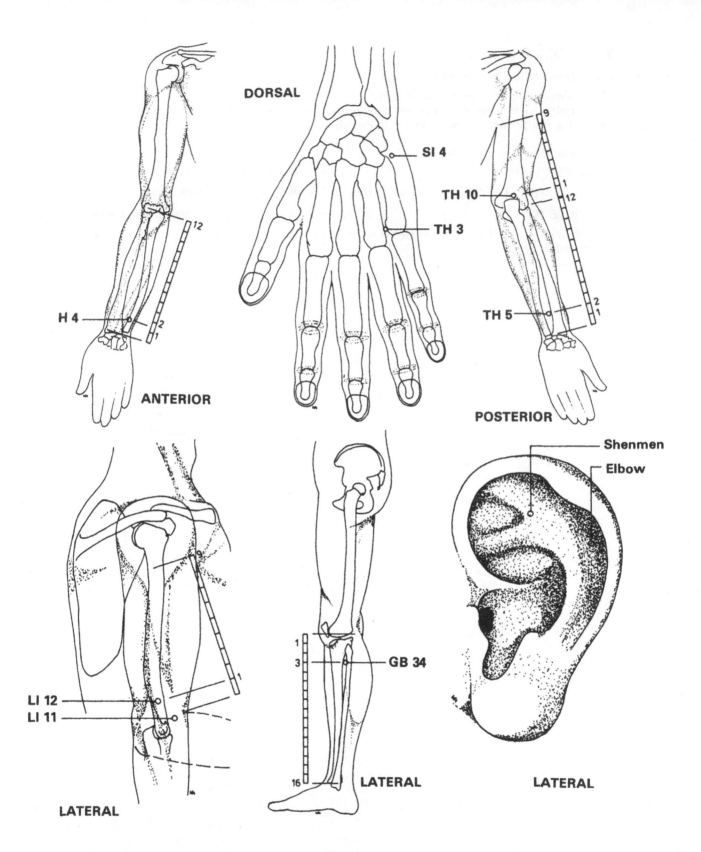

DORSAL

SI 4

TH 3

ANTERIOR

H 4

12

2

1

POSTERIOR

TH 10

TH 5

9

1

12

2

1

LATERAL

LI 12

LI 11

LATERAL

GB 34

1

3

16

LATERAL

Shenmen

Elbow

LATERAL

82

ELBOW PAIN

Choose from the following points:

Meridian	Point Ref	Chinese Name	Anatomical Position	Depth of Insertion (inches)	Special Note
LARGE INTESTINE	LI 11	Ch'ü Ch'ih	With the forearm flexed to a 90° angle, this point lies between lateral epicondyle and lateral edge of elbow fold.	1	
LARGE INTESTINE	LI 12	Chou Liao	With the arm as above, this point is 1 AUM proximal to Chü Ch'ih. On lateral border of humerus.	1	
TRIPLE HEATER	TH 10	T'ien Ching	1 AUM proximal to olecrenon process.	¾	
GALL BLADDER	GB 34	Yang Ling Ch'üan	In the depression antero-inferior to small head of fibula.	1¼	

Ah Shi (local spontaneously tender) points are useful.

Auricular Points

ELBOW POINT			In scapha, level with superior border of concha.		
EAR SHENMEN POINT			In inferior corner of bifurcating point of antihelix.		

For arthritic pain of elbow, add:

Meridian	Point Ref	Chinese Name	Anatomical Position	Depth of Insertion (inches)	Special Note
HEART	H 4	Ling Tao	1½ AUM proximal to wrist crease on radial side of flexor carpi ulnaris.	½	
SMALL INTESTINE	SI 4	Wan Ku	Ulna aspects of palm, proximal to base of 5th metacarpal.	¼	
TRIPLE HEATER	TH 3	Chung Chu	Dorsal surface of hand, proximal and between heads of 4th and 5th metacarpals.	½	
TRIPLE HEATER	TH 5	Wai Kuan	2 AUM proximal to dorsal wrist crease between radius and ulna.	¾	

Treatment should consist of strong stimulation which can be combined with moxibustion unless otherwise indicated.

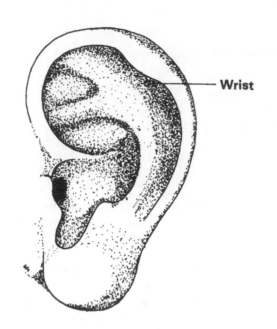

Wrist

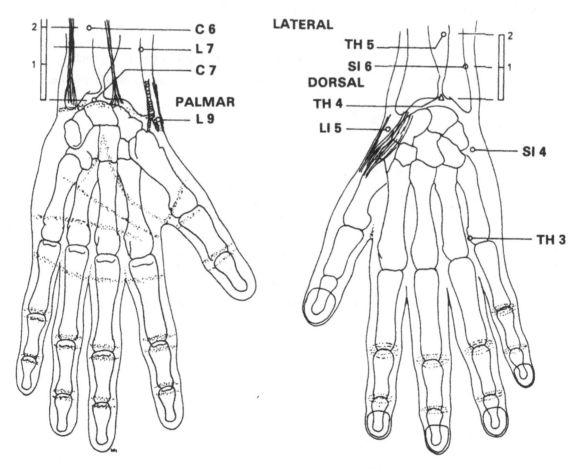

2
1
C 6
L 7
C 7
PALMAR
L 9

LATERAL
TH 5
SI 6
2
1
DORSAL
TH 4
LI 5
SI 4
TH 3

WRIST PAIN

Choose from:

Meridian	Point Ref	Chinese Name	Anatomical Position	Depth of Insertion (inches)	Special Note
LARGE INTESTINE	LI 5	Yang Ch'i	Radial aspect of dorsum of wrist; with thumb hyper-extended, it lies in depression between tendons of extensor pollicis longus and brevis.	¼	
TRIPLE HEATER	TH 4	Yang Ch'ih	In depression at centre of dorsal surface of wrist.	¼	Cauterization forbidden.
TRIPLE HEATER	TH 5	Wai Kuan	2 AUM proximal to dorsal wrist crease between radius and ulna.	½	
LUNG	L 9	T'ai Yüan	Between abductor pollicis longus and radial artery. On palmer surface of wrist.	¼	Avoid artery
LUNG	L 7	Lieh Ch'üeh	1½ AUM proximal to transverse wrist crease above styloid process of radius.	½	Needle insertion obliquely upwards.

For stenosing tenosynovitis (de Quervains disease), add:

Ah Shi (local spontaneously tender) points.

For compression of median nerve at wrist, add:

CIRCULATION	C 6	Nei Kuan	2 AUM above wrist crease, between tendons of palmaris longus and flexor carpi radialis.	¾	
CIRCULATION	C 7	Ta Ling	Midpoint of transverse wrist crease, between tendons of palmaris longus and flexor carpi radialis.	¾	

For 'wrist drop', add:

SMALL INTESTINE	SI 6	Yang Lao	On dorsum of forearm 1 AUM proximal to styloid process of ulna.	1	

Auricular Point

WRIST POINT   In scapha, level with superior aspect of deltoid fossa.

continued overleaf

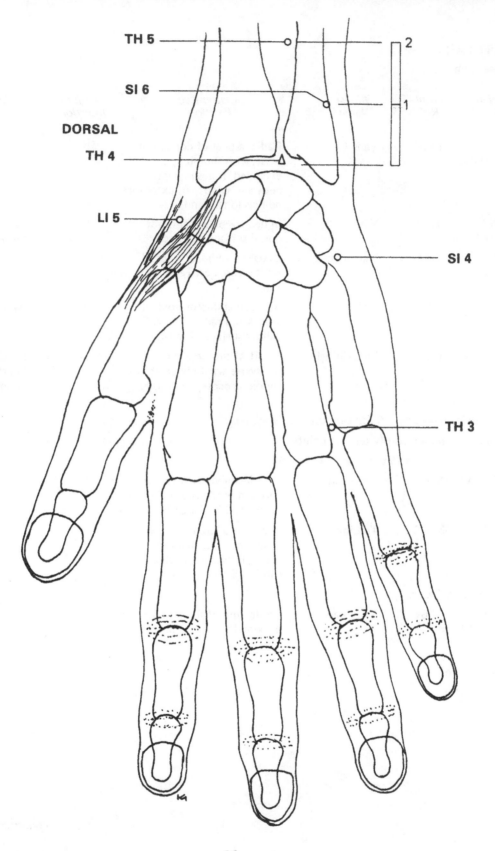

TH 5

SI 6

2

1

DORSAL

TH 4

LI 5

SI 4

TH 3

WRIST PAIN (contd.)

Meridian	Point Ref	Chinese Name	Anatomical Position	Depth of Insertion (inches)	Special Note
For arthritic pain, add:					
SMALL INTESTINE	SI 4	Wan Ku	Ulna aspect of palm, proximal to base of 5th metacarpal.	¼	
TRIPLE HEATER	TH 3	Chung Chu	Dorsal surface of hand proximal, and between, heads of 4th and 5th metacarpals.	½	
TRIPLE HEATER	TH 4	Yang Ch'ih	In depression at centre of dorsal surface of wrist.	½	Cauterization forbidden.

No more than 5 or 6 points should be used at any treatment. Moxibustion is useful in these conditions (unless points are indicated as forbidden).

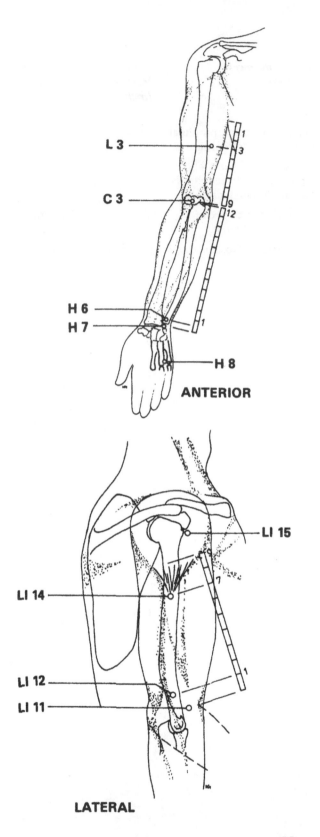

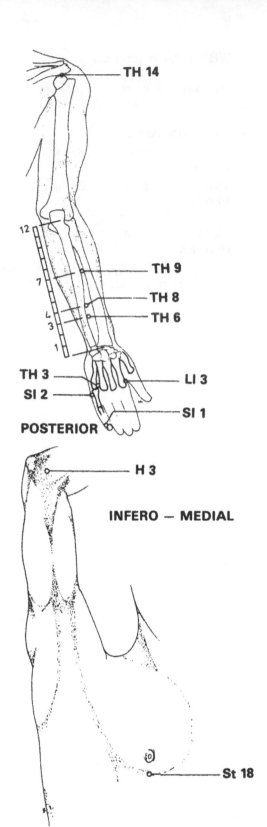

L 3

C 3

H 6

H 7

H 8

ANTERIOR

TH 14

TH 9

TH 8

TH 6

TH 3

SI 2

LI 3

SI 1

POSTERIOR

LI 15

LI 14

LI 12

LI 11

LATERAL

H 3

INFERO — MEDIAL

St 18

ARM
Neuralgia (Intermittent Pain)

Choose 5 or 6 points at each treatment from the following:

Meridian	Point Ref	Chinese Name	Anatomical Position	Depth of Insertion (inches)	Special Note
HEART	H 8	Shao Fu	Palm of hand, between 4th and 5th metacarpals on distal palm crease.	¼	
CIRCULATION	C 3	Chü Chih	Centre of elbow crease. Ulna side of tendon of biceps.	¾	
TRIPLE HEATER	TH 3	Chung Chu	Dorsal surface of hand proximal and between heads of 4th and 5th metacarpals.	½	
TRIPLE HEATER	TH 6	Chih Kou	Posterior surface of forearm between radius and ulna, 3 AUM proximal to wrist crease.	¾	
TRIPLE HEATER	TH 8	San Yang Lê	1 AUM proximal to Chih Kou	¾	
TRIPLE HEATER	TH 9	Ssŭ Tu	7 AUM proximal to wrist crease, between radius and ulna.	¾	
TRIPLE HEATER	TH 14	Chien Liao	Dorsal surface of shoulder between acromion and greater tubercle of humerus.	1¼	With arm raised horizontally, insert needle between acromion and tubercle towards axilla.
LUNG	L 3	T'ien Fu	Medial aspect of upper arm 3 AUM below anterior axillary fold.	¾	
LARGE INTESTINE	LI 3	San Chien	Radial aspect of index finger proximal to head of metacarpal bone.	½	
LARGE INTESTINE	LI 11	Ch'u Ch'ih	Lateral aspect of elbow crease between lateral epicondyle and edge of elbow fold.	1	
LARGE INTESTINE	LI 12	Chou Liao	1 AUM proximal to Ch'ü Ch'ih on lateral border of humerus.	1	
LARGE INTESTINE	LI 14	Pi Nao	External aspect of arm 7 AUM above elbow crease at distal end of deltoid muscle.	½–1	
LARGE INTESTINE	LI 15	Chien Yü	Antero-inferior aspect of acromio-clavicular joint.	¾–1	

continued overleaf

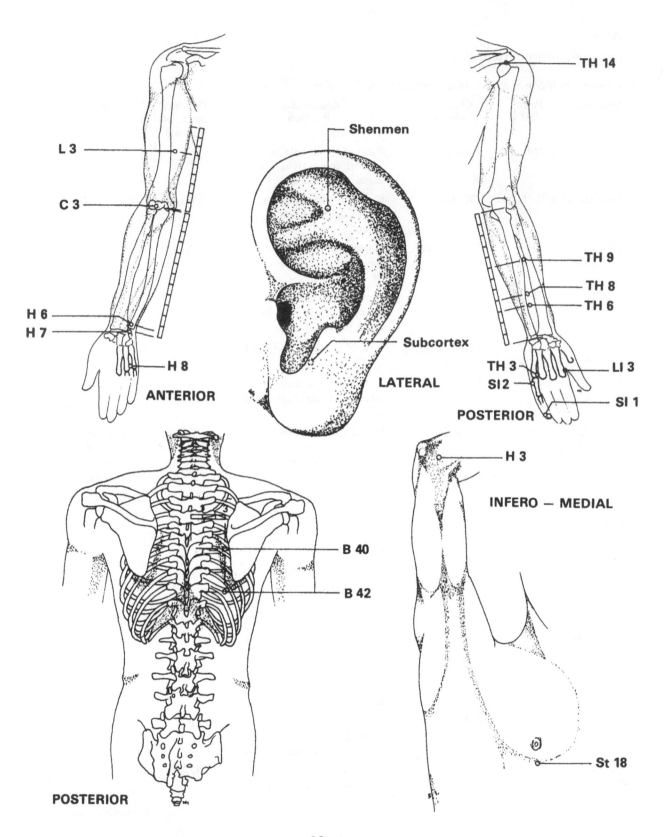

L 3

C 3

H 6
H 7

H 8

ANTERIOR

Shenmen

Subcortex

LATERAL

TH 14

TH 9

TH 8
TH 6

TH 3
SI2

LI 3

SI 1

POSTERIOR

B 40

B 42

POSTERIOR

H 3

INFERO — MEDIAL

St 18

ARM
Neuralgia (Intermittent Pain) (contd.)

Meridian	Point Ref	Chinese Name	Anatomical Position	Depth of Insertion (inches)	Special Note
STOMACH	St 18	Ju Ken	In 5th intercostal space, below nipple.	½	Oblique insertion.
SMALL INTESTINE	SI 1	Shao Chih	On little finger just proximal to lateral nail root.	$\frac{1}{10}$	
SMALL INTESTINE	SI 2	Ch'ien Ku	In depression distal to outer aspect of 5th metacarpo-phalangeal joint.	¼	

If forearm is more involved, add:

Meridian	Point Ref	Chinese Name	Anatomical Position	Depth of Insertion (inches)	Special Note
HEART	H3	Shao Hai	Internal aspect of flexure of elbow.	¾	
HEART	H 6	Yin Ch'i	½ AUM proximal to wrist crease, radial side of tendon of flexor carpi ulnaris.	½	
HEART	H 7	Shen Men	Ulna aspect of wrist, on proximal border of pisiform bone, in a depression.	½	

If axilla is involved, add:

Meridian	Point Ref	Chinese Name	Anatomical Position	Depth of Insertion (inches)	Special Note
BLADDER	B 40[1]	I Hsi	3 AUM lateral to lower end of 6th thoracic spinous process.	¼—½	
BLADDER	B 42[2]	Hun Men	3 AUM lateral to lower end of 9th thoracic spinous process.	¼—½	

Auricular Points

EAR SHENMEN POINT	Inferior corner of bifurcating point of antihelix.
SUBCORTEX POINT	Interior wall of antitragus.

[1] Recent Chinese texts show this as Bladder 45.
[2] Recent Chinese texts show this as Bladder 47.

DORSAL

Shang
Pa Hsieh

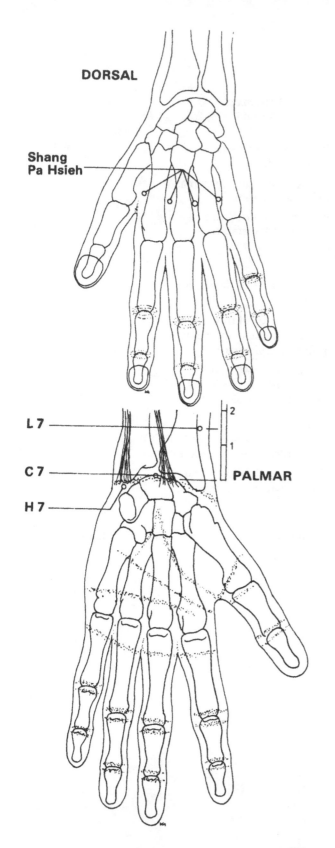

L 7

C 7

PALMAR

H 7

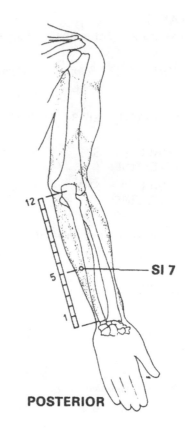

12

5

SI 7

1

POSTERIOR

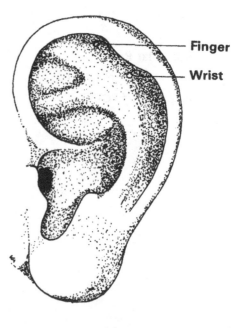

Finger

Wrist

LATERAL

HAND AND FINGER PAIN

Meridian	Point Ref	Chinese Name	Anatomical Position	Depth of Insertion (inches)	Special Note
SMALL INTESTINE	SI 7	Chih Cheng	5 AUM proximal to wrist on postero-medial aspect of forearm, just medial to ulna.	¾	
SHANG PA HSIEH POINTS			These lie on dorsal surface of hand in web between distal portions of metacarpals. There are 4 such points on each hand. (The point between 1st and 2nd metacarpals is Ho Ku, Large Intestine 4).	¾	Insert needle obliquely cephalidward.

For pain in the ring or little finger, add:

Meridian	Point Ref	Chinese Name	Anatomical Position	Depth of Insertion (inches)	Special Note
HEART	H 7	Shen Men	Ulna aspect of wrist, on proximal border of pisiform bone, in a depression.	½	

For pain in the index or middle finger, add:

Meridian	Point Ref	Chinese Name	Anatomical Position	Depth of Insertion (inches)	Special Note
CIRCULATION	C 7	Ta Ling	Midpoint of tranverse wrist crease between tendons of palmaris longus and flexor carpi radialis.	¼	

For thumb pain, add:

Meridian	Point Ref	Chinese Name	Anatomical Position	Depth of Insertion (inches)	Special Note
LUNG	L 7	Lieh Ch'üeh	1½ AUM proximal to transverse wrist crease, above styloid process of radius.	½	Needle insertion obliquely upwards.

Auricular Points

FINGER POINT — Superior aspect of scapha.

WRIST POINT — In scapha level with superior aspect of deltoid fossa.

DORSAL

LI 4

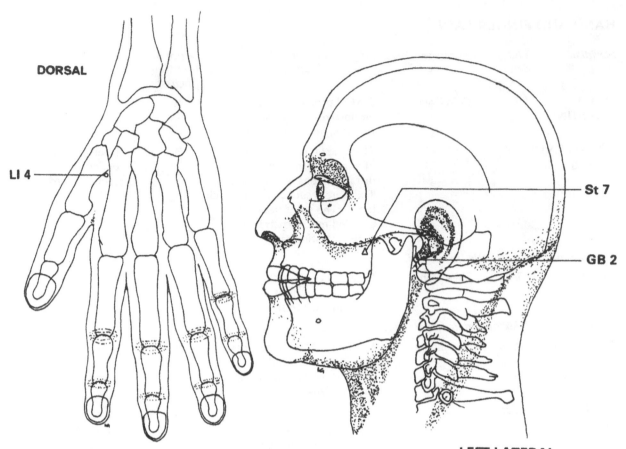

St 7

GB 2

LEFT LATERAL

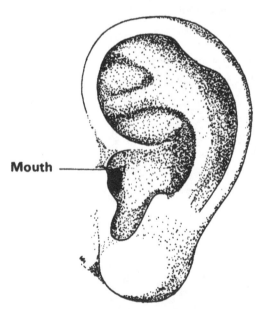

Mouth

LATERAL

94

JAW
General Pain

Meridian	Point Ref	Chinese Name	Anatomical Position	Depth of Insertion (inches)	Special Note
LARGE INTESTINE	LI 4	Ho Ku	Dorsal surface of hand in angle of first 2 metacarpals.	1	
STOMACH	St 7	Hsia Kuan	Anterior to head of mandible in infratemporal fossa.	¾	Cauterization forbidden.
GALL BLADDER	GB 2	T'ing Hui	Anterior to lobe of ear, posterior to condyle of mandible.	1	

Auricular Points

MOUTH POINT   Close to posterior wall of external auditory meatus.

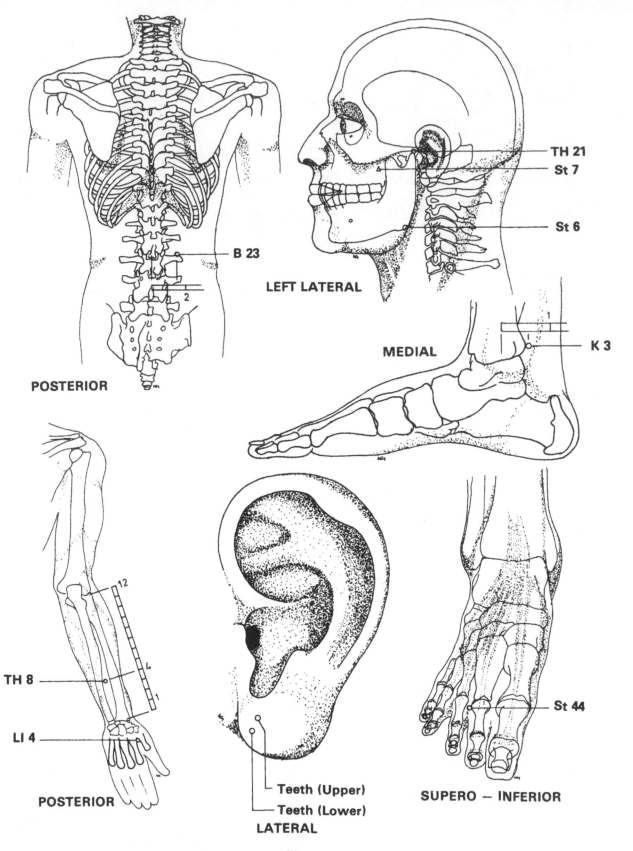

POSTERIOR

B 23

LEFT LATERAL

TH 21
St 7
St 6

MEDIAL

K 3

TH 8

LI 4

POSTERIOR

Teeth (Upper)
Teeth (Lower)

LATERAL

SUPERO — INFERIOR

St 44

TOOTHACHE
of Upper Jaw

Meridian	Point Ref	Chinese Name	Anatomical Position	Depth of Insertion (inches)	Special Note
LARGE INTESTINE	LI 4	Ho Ku	Dorsal surface of hand in angle of 1st 2 metacarpals.	1	Strong stimulation for 3 or 4 minutes.
STOMACH	St 7	Hsia Kuan	Anterior to head of mandible in infratemporal fossa.	¾	Cauterization forbidden.
TRIPLE HEATER	TH 21	Erh Men	Anterior to ear, slightly superior to condyle of mandible.	¾	Insert needle with mouth open.

of Lower Jaw

Meridian	Point Ref	Chinese Name	Anatomical Position	Depth of Insertion (inches)	Special Note
LARGE INTESTINE	LI 4	Ho Ku	Dorsal surface of hand in angle of 1st 2 metacarpals.	1	Strong stimulation for 3 or 4 minutes.
STOMACH	St 6	Chia Ch'ê	At angle of Jaw between insertions of masseter muscle.	1 ¼	Towards corner of mouth *or* perpendicularly.
TRIPLE HEATER	TH 8	San Yang Lê	Posterior forearm, 4 AUM above wrist crease between radius and ulna.	¾	Some authorities ban the needling of this point and recommend cauterization.

Also useful in toothache are:

Meridian	Point Ref	Chinese Name	Anatomical Position	Depth of Insertion (inches)	Special Note
STOMACH	St 44	Nei T'ing	Dorsal surface of foot ½ AUM proximal to web between 2nd and 3rd toes.	½	
KIDNEY	K 3	T'ai Ch'i	Internal aspect of foot ½ AUM posterior to malleolus.	½	
BLADDER	B 23	Shen Yü	1½ AUM lateral to median line at level of interspace between 2nd and 3rd lumbar vertebrae.	1	

Auricular Points

TEETH (UPPER) POINT — On the ear-lobe above and behind 'Teeth (Lower) Point'.

TEETH (LOWER) POINT — On the ear-lobe (see auricle diagram).

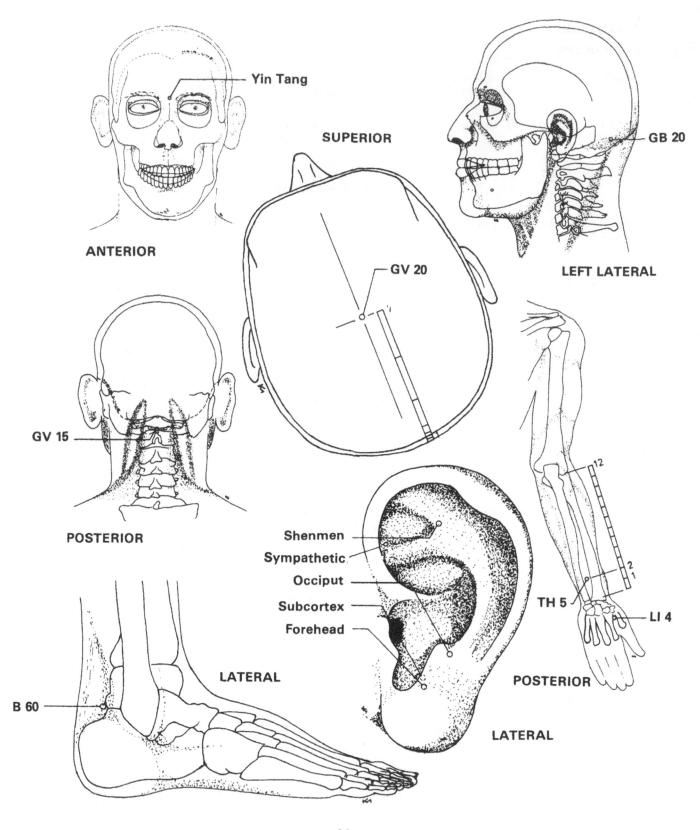

Yin Tang

ANTERIOR

SUPERIOR

GB 20

LEFT LATERAL

GV 20

GV 15

POSTERIOR

Shenmen
Sympathetic
Occiput
Subcortex
Forehead

12

2
1

TH 5

LI 4

POSTERIOR

LATERAL

B 60

LATERAL

HEADACHE
General

Only mild stimulation should be given to points on the head. The needles should be left *in situ* for up to 20 minutes.

Meridian	Point Ref	Chinese Name	Anatomical Position	Depth of Insertion (inches)	Special Note
GOVERNOR VESSEL	GV 15	Ya Men	½ AUM above hairline between processes of 1st and 2nd cervical vertebrae.	1	Head held slightly forward, insert slowly towards mandible. Do not manipulate needle.
LARGE INTESTINE	LI 4	Ho Ku	Dorsal surface of hand in angle of 1st 2 metacarpals.	1	
TRIPLE HEATER	TH 5	Wai Kuan	Posterior surface of forearm between radius and ulna, 2 AUM proximal to dorsal crease.	¾	
EXTRA 1		Yin Tang	On the glabella.	½	Horizontally downwards just under the skin.
BLADDER	B 60	Kun Lun	Lateral surface of ankle, between external malleolus and Achilles tendon. Level with prominence of malleolus.	¾	
GALL BLADDER	GB 20	Fêng Ch'ih	Between depression inferior to occipital protuberance, and mastoid bone.	1	Needle towards orbit on opposite side, no deeper than indicated.
GOVERNOR VESSEL	GV 20	Pai Hui	On vertex of skull, 7 AUM above posterior hairline, on a line connecting apex of ears.	¼	Posteriorly.

Auricular Points

OCCIPUT POINT	Posterior and superior to lateral aspect of antitragus.
FOREHEAD POINT	Anterior and inferior to lateral side of antitragus.
SYMPATHETIC NERVE POINT	In deltoid fossa at junction of infra-antihelix crus and medial border of helix.
EAR SHENMEN POINT	In inferior corner of bifurcating point of antihelix.
SUBCORTEX POINT	Interior wall of antitragus.

99

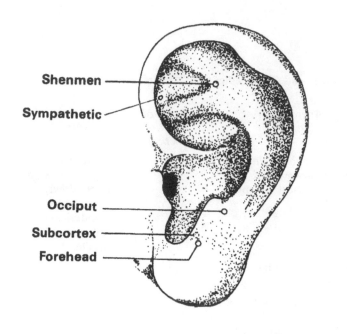

Shenmen

Sympathetic

Occiput

Subcortex

Forehead

LATERAL

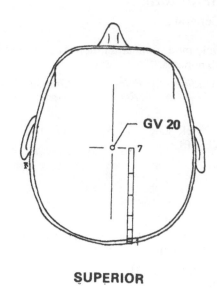

GV 20

7

SUPERIOR

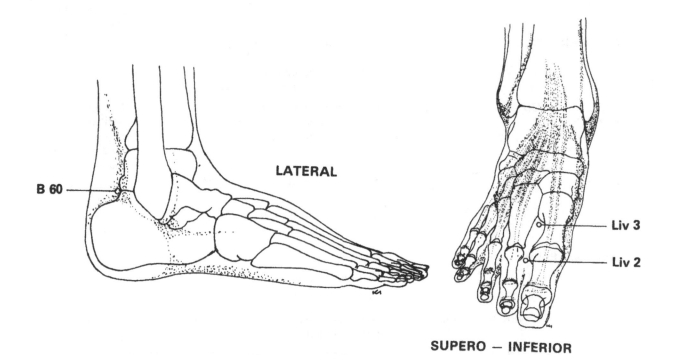

B 60

LATERAL

Liv 3

Liv 2

SUPERO — INFERIOR

HEADACHE

Vertex

Only mild stimulation should be given to points on the head. The needles should be left *in situ* for up to 20 minutes.

Meridian	Point Ref	Chinese Name	Anatomical Position	Depth of Insertion (inches)	Special Note
GOVERNOR VESSEL	GV 20	Pai Hui	On vertex of skull, 7 AUM above posterior hairline on a line connecting apex of ears.	¼	Posteriorly
BLADDER	B 60	Kun Lun	Lateral surface of ankle, between external malleolus and Achilles tendon. Level with prominence of malleolus.	¾	
LIVER	Liv 2	Hsing Chien	½ AUM proximal to web margin between 1st and 2nd toes.	¼	
LIVER	Liv 3	T'ai Ch'ung	On dorsal surface of foot in angle between 1st and 2nd metatarsals.	¼	

Auricular Points

OCCIPUT POINT	Posterior and superior to lateral aspect of antitragus.
FOREHEAD POINT	Anterior and inferior to lateral side of antitragus.
SYMPATHETIC NERVE POINT	In deltoid fossa at junction of infra-antihelix crus and medial border of helix.
SUBCORTEX POINT	Interior wall of antitragus.
EAR SHENMEN POINT	In inferior corner of bifurcating point of antihelix.

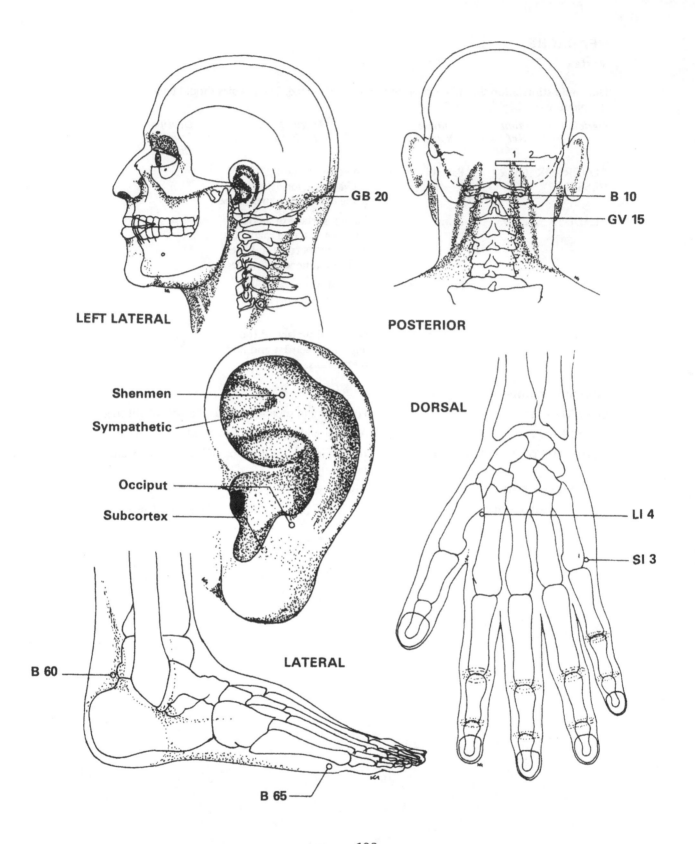

LEFT LATERAL

GB 20

POSTERIOR

B 10

GV 15

Shenmen

Sympathetic

Occiput

Subcortex

DORSAL

LI 4

SI 3

LATERAL

B 60

B 65

102

HEADACHE
Occipital

Only mild stimulation should be given to points on the head. The needles should be left *in situ* for up to 20 minutes.

Meridian	Point Ref	Chinese Name	Anatomical Position	Depth of Insertion (inches)	Special Note
GALL BLADDER	GB 20	Fêng Ch'ih	Between depression inferior to occipital protuberance, and mastoid bone.	1	Needle towards opposite orbit, no deeper than indicated.
GOVERNOR VESSEL	GV 15	Ya Men	½ AUM above hairline between processes of 1st and 2nd cervicle vertebrae.	1	With head held slightly forward, insert slowly towards mandible. Do not manipulate needle.
BLADDER	B 10	T'ien Chu	Posterior neck. 1½ AUM lateral to midline, level with interspace between 1st and 2nd cervical vertebrae.	¾	
BLADDER	B 60	Kun Lun	Lateral surface of ankle, between external malleolus and Achilles tendon. Level with prominence of malleolus.	¾	
LARGE INTESTINE	LI 4	Ho Ku	Dorsal surface of hand in angle of 1st 2 metacarpals.	1	
SMALL INTESTINE	SI 3	Hou Ch'i	Just proximal to metacarpo-phalangeal articulation of little finger.	¼	
BLADDER	B 65	Shu Ku	External aspect of foot behind metatarso-phalangeal joint of 5th toe.	¼	

Auricular Points

OCCIPUT POINT — Posterior and superior to lateral aspect of antitragus.

SYMPATHETIC NERVE POINT — In deltoid fossa at junction of infra-antihelix crus and medial border of helix.

EAR SHENMEN POINT — In inferior corner of bifurcating point of antihelix.

SUBCORTEX POINT — Interior wall of antitragus.

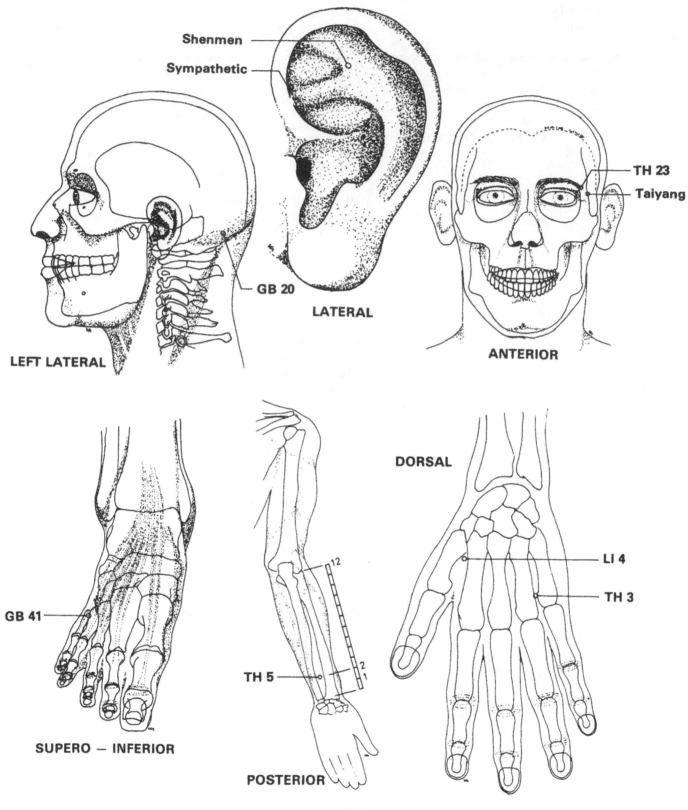

Shenmen

Sympathetic

GB 20

LATERAL

LEFT LATERAL

TH 23

Taiyang

ANTERIOR

DORSAL

GB 41

LI 4

TH 3

SUPERO — INFERIOR

TH 5

POSTERIOR

104

HEADACHE
Temporal

Only mild stimulation should be given to points on the head. The needles should be left *in situ* for up to 20 minutes.

Meridian	Point Ref	Chinese Name	Anatomical Position	Depth of Insertion (inches)	Special Note
LARGE INTESTINE	LI 4	Ho Ku	Dorsal surface of hand in angle between 1st 2 metacarpals.	1	
TRIPLE HEATER	TH 23	Ssŭ Chu K'ung	Lateral margin of eyebrow.	½	Insert needle horizontally posteriorly.
TRIPLE HEATER	TH 5	Wai Kuan	Posterior surface of forearm between radius and ulna, 2 AUM proximal to dorsal crease.	¾	
EXTRA 2		Taiyang	In a depression 1 AUM posterior posterior to midpoint between lateral eyebrow margin and outer canthus.	½ or 1	Perpendicularly or obliquely downwards.
GALL BLADDER	GB 20	Fêng Ch'ih	Between depression inferior to occipital protuberance, and mastoid bone.	1	Needle towards orbit on opposite side. No deeper than indicated.
GALL BLADDER	GB 41	(Tsu) Lin Ch'i	In depression distal to junction of 4th and 5th metatarsal bones.	¾	
TRIPLE HEATER	TH 3	Ch'ung Chu	Dorsal surface of hand between 4th and 5th metacarpals, slightly proximal to metacarpo-phalangeal joint.	½	

Auricular Points

SYMPATHETIC NERVE POINT   In deltoid fossa at junction of infra-antihelix crus and medial border of helix.

EAR SHENMEN POINT   In inferior corner of bifurcating point of antihelix.

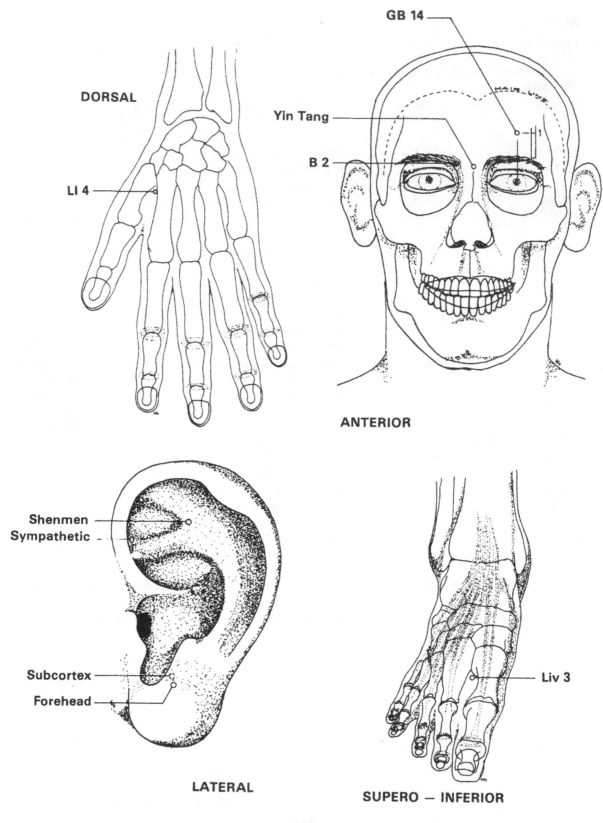

DORSAL

LI 4

GB 14

Yin Tang

B 2

ANTERIOR

Shenmen
Sympathetic

Subcortex

Forehead

LATERAL

Liv 3

SUPERO — INFERIOR

106

HEADACHE
Frontal

Only mild stimulation should be given to points on the head. The needles should be left *in situ* for up to 20 minutes.

Meridian	Point Ref	Chinese Name	Anatomical Position	Depth of Insertion (inches)	Special Note
EXTRA 1		Yin Tang	On the glabella.	½	Horizontally downwards just under skin.
GALL BLADDER	GB 14	Yang Pai	On forehead, 1 AUM proximal to eyebrow, directly above pupil.	½	Horizontally inferiorly.
LARGE INTESTINE	LI 4	Ho Ku	Dorsal surface of hand in angle of 1st 2 metacarpals.	1	
BLADDER	B 2	Ts'uan Chu	At medial margin of eyebrow.	¼	
LIVER	Liv 3	T'ai Ch'ung	Between 1st and 2nd toes 2 AUM proximal to margin of web.	¾	Obliquely upwards.

Auricular Points

FOREHEAD POINT	Anterior and inferior to lateral side of antitragus.
SYMPATHETIC NERVE POINT	In deltoid fossa at junction of infra-antihelix crus and medial border of helix.
SUBCORTEX POINT	Interior wall of antitragus.
EAR SHENMEN POINT	In inferior corner of bifurcating point of antihelix.

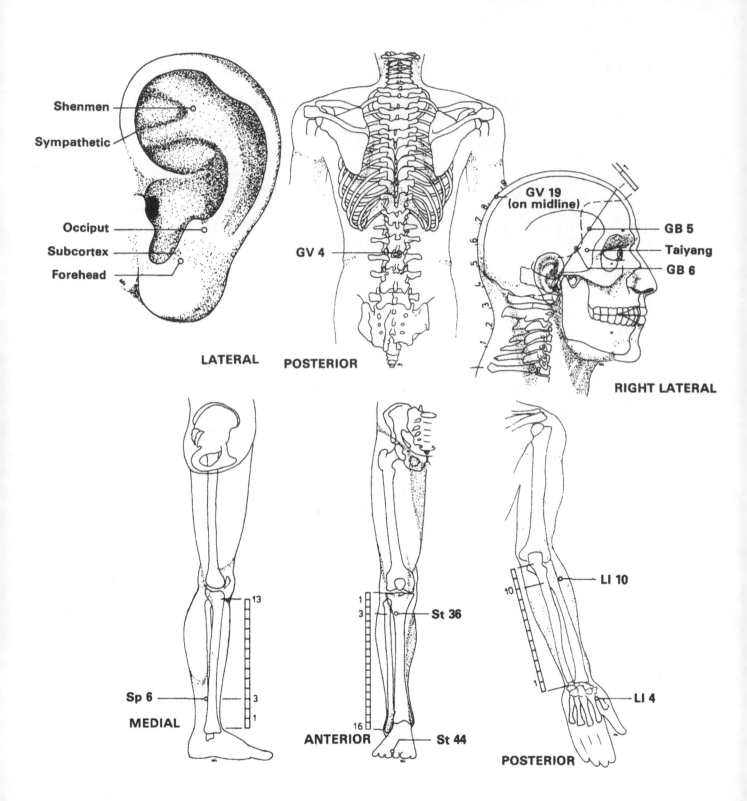

Shenmen

Sympathetic

Occiput

Subcortex

Forehead

LATERAL

GV 4

POSTERIOR

GV 19
(on midline)

GB 5

Taiyang

GB 6

RIGHT LATERAL

13

Sp 6

3

1

MEDIAL

1

3

St 36

16

ANTERIOR

St 44

10

LI 10

1

LI 4

POSTERIOR

108

HEADACHE
Migraine

Meridian	Point Ref	Chinese Name	Anatomical Position	Depth of Insertion (inches)	Special Note
GALL BLADDER	GB 5	Hsüan Lu	Located upon temple. Halfway along a line between external auditory meatus and a point on midline, ½ AUM above anterior hairline.	¼	
GALL BLADDER	GB 6	Hsüan Li	Located 1 AUM inferior to GB 5 on same line as above.	¼	
LARGE INTESTINE	LI 4	Ho Ku	Dorsal surface of hand in angle between 1st 2 metacarpals.	1	
LARGE INTESTINE	LI 10	(Shou) San Li	Dorsal surface of forearm 2 AUM distal to radial extremity of elbow flexure.	1	
STOMACH	St 36	(Tsu) San Li	3 AUM distal to knee crease, 1 finger's width lateral to anterior crest of tibia.	1¼	
STOMACH	St 44	Nei T'ing	½ AUM proximal to web margin between 2nd and 3rd toes.	¼	
SPLEEN	Sp 6	San Yin Chiao	3 AUM[1] proximal to prominence of medial malleolus, posterior to tibial border.	1	
GOVERNOR VESSEL	GV 4	Ming Men	On the midline between spinous processes of 2nd and 3rd lumbar vertebrae.	1	Needle tilted slightly upwards.
GOVERNOR VESSEL	GV 19	Hou Ting	On midline 8½ AUM proximal to lower border of spinous process of 7th cervical vertebra.	¾	Obliquely.
EXTRA 2		Taiyang	In a depression 1 AUM posterior to midpoint between lateral eyebrow margin and outer canthus.	½	

Auricular Points

OCCIPUT POINT	Posterior and superior to lateral aspect of antitragus.
FOREHEAD POINT	Anterior and inferior to lateral aspect of antitragus.
SYMPATHETIC NERVE POINT	In deltoid fossa at junction of infra-antihelix crus and medial border of helix.
EAR SHENMEN POINT	In inferior corner of bifurcating point of antihelix.
SUBCORTEX POINT	Interior wall of antitragus.

[1] Note some Western authorities give this as 4 AUM.

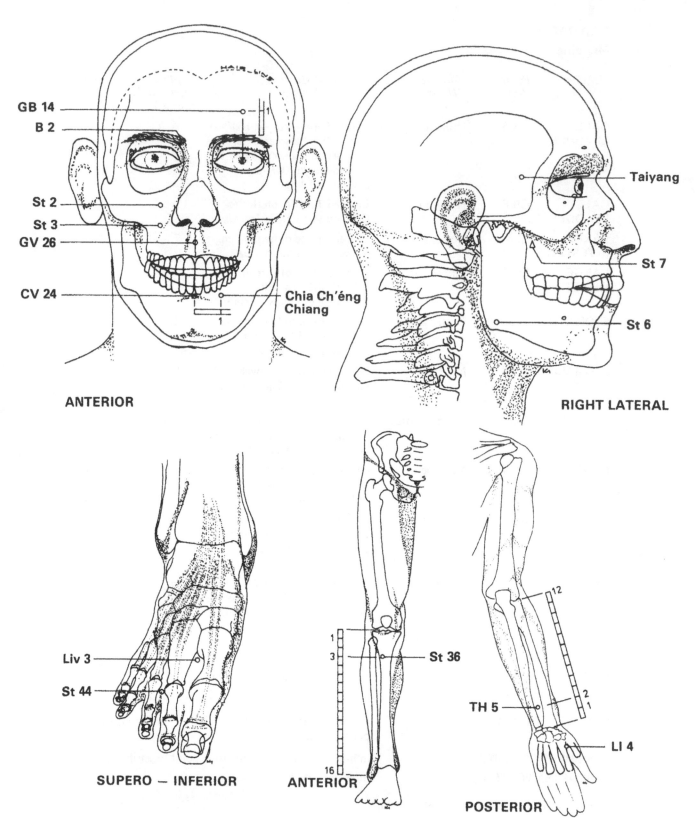

GB 14

B 2

St 2

St 3

GV 26

CV 24

Chia Ch'éng
Chiang

ANTERIOR

Taiyang

St 7

St 6

RIGHT LATERAL

Liv 3

St 44

SUPERO — INFERIOR

St 36

ANTERIOR

TH 5

LI 4

POSTERIOR

110

TRIGEMINAL NEURALGIA

Treatment of distant points should be vigorous and treatment of local points mild. Needles should be left *in situ* for up to 40 minutes, with periodic stimulation. Distal points should be selected according to meridian pathways. Choose 3 or 4 points at each treatment.

Opthalmic (first) Division

Meridian	Point Ref	Chinese Name	Anatomical Position	Depth of Insertion (inches)	Special Note
GALL BLADDER	GB 14	Yang Pai	On forehead, 1 AUM proximal to eyebrow, directly above pupil.	½	Horizontally inferiorly.
BLADDER	B 2	Tsuan Chu	Medial margin of eyebrow.	¼—½	Subcutaneously down or lateral.
TRIPLE HEATER	TH 5	Wai Kuan	Posterior surface of forearm between radius and ulna 2 AUM proximal to dorsal crease.	¾	
EXTRA 2		Taiyang	In a depression 1 AUM posterior to midpoint between lateral end of eyebrow and outer canthus.	½ or 1	Perpendicularly or obliquely downwards.
STOMACH	St 2	Ssŭ Pai	In infraorbital foramen ¾ AUM directly below infraorbital margin.	¼	
STOMACH	St 7	Hsia Kuan	Anterior to head of mandible in infratemporal fossa.	¾	Cauterization forbidden.
EXTRA 5		Chia Ch'êng Chiang	1 AUM lateral to depression between point of chin and lower lip.	¼	
STOMACH	St 44	Nei T'ing	Dorsal aspect of foot. ½ AUM proximal to web margin between 2nd and 3rd metatarsals.	½	Obliquely upwards.
LIVER	Liv 3	T'ai Ch'ung	Between 1st and 2nd metatarsals, 2 AUM proximal to metatarso-phalangeal joints.	¾	Obliquely upwards
STOMACH	St 36	(Tsu) San Li	3 AUM inferior to knee crease, 1 finger's width lateral to crest of tibia.	1—1½	
LARGE INTESTINE	LI 4	Ho Ku	Dorsal surface of hand in angle of 1st 2 metacarpals.	1	

Maxillary (second) Division

Meridian	Point Ref	Chinese Name	Anatomical Position	Depth of Insertion (inches)	Special Note
STOMACH	St 2	Ssŭ Pai	In infraorbital foramen ¾ AUM directly below infraorbital margin.	¼	

continued overleaf

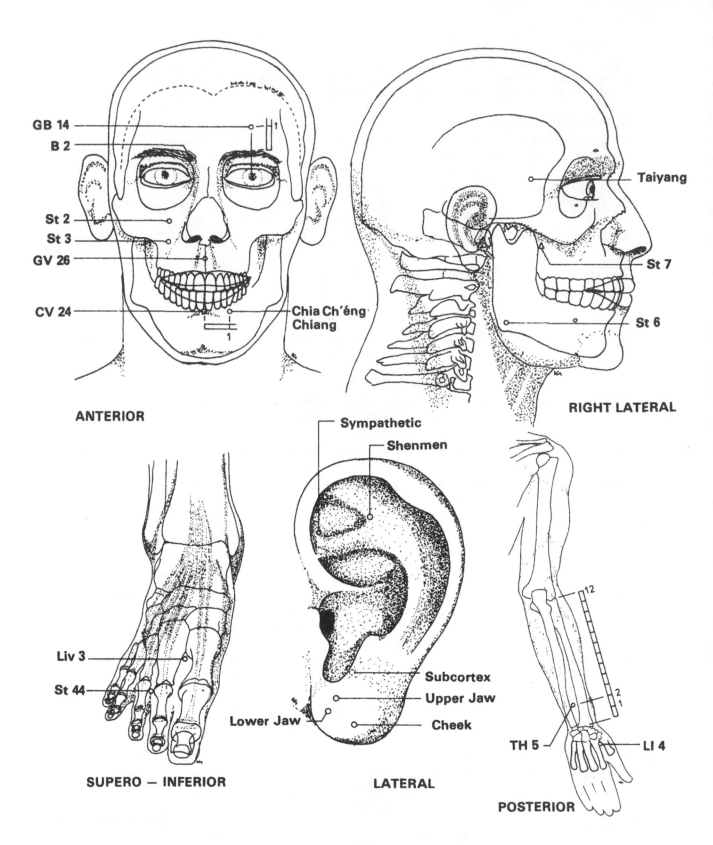

GB 14

B 2

St 2

St 3

GV 26

CV 24

Chia Ch'éng
Chiang

ANTERIOR

Taiyang

St 7

St 6

RIGHT LATERAL

Liv 3

St 44

SUPERO — INFERIOR

Sympathetic

Shenmen

Subcortex

Upper Jaw

Lower Jaw

Cheek

LATERAL

TH 5

LI 4

POSTERIOR

112

TRIGEMINAL NEURALGIA (contd.)

Meridian	Point Ref	Chinese Name	Anatomical Position	Depth of Insertion (inches)	Special Note
GOVERNOR VESSEL	GV 26	Shui Kou	On median line of face, below nose; centre of philtrum.	¼	Needle slightly upwards
LARGE INTESTINE	LI 4	Ho Ku	Dorsal surface of hand in angle of 1st 2 metacarpals.	1	
STOMACH	St 3	Chü Liao	Directly below Stomach 2 at level of lower end of ala nasi, lateral to groove.	½	
STOMACH	St 44	Nei T'ing	Dorsal aspect of foot ½ AUM proximal to web margin between 2nd and 3rd metatarsals.	½	Obliquely upwards.

Mandibular (third) Division

Meridian	Point Ref	Chinese Name	Anatomical Position	Depth of Insertion (inches)	Special Note
STOMACH	St 7	Hsia Kuan	Anterior to head of mandible in infratemporal fossa.	¾	Cauterization forbidden.
EXTRA 5		Chia Ch'êng Chiang	1 AUM lateral to depression between point of chin and lower lip.	¼	
STOMACH	St 6	Chia Ch'ê	Anterior and superior to angle of jaw on prominence of masseter muscle.	1 or ¼	Towards corner of mouth or perpendicularly.
CONCEPTION VESSEL	CV 24	Ch'êng Chiang	On medial line of face in depression between point of chin and lower lip.	¼	
STOMACH	St 44	Nei T'ing	Dorsal aspect of foot ½ AUM proximal to web margin between 2nd and 3rd metatarsals.	½	Obliquely upwards.

Auricular Points

SYMPATHETIC POINT	In deltoid fossa at junction of infra-antihelix crus and medial border of helix.
EAR SHENMEN POINT	In inferior corner of bifurcating point of antihelix.
SUBCORTEX POINT	Interior wall of antitragus.
CHEEK POINT	Infero-central area of ear-lobe.
LOWER JAW POINT	In central superior area of ear-lobe.
UPPER JAW POINT	In central area of ear-lobe.

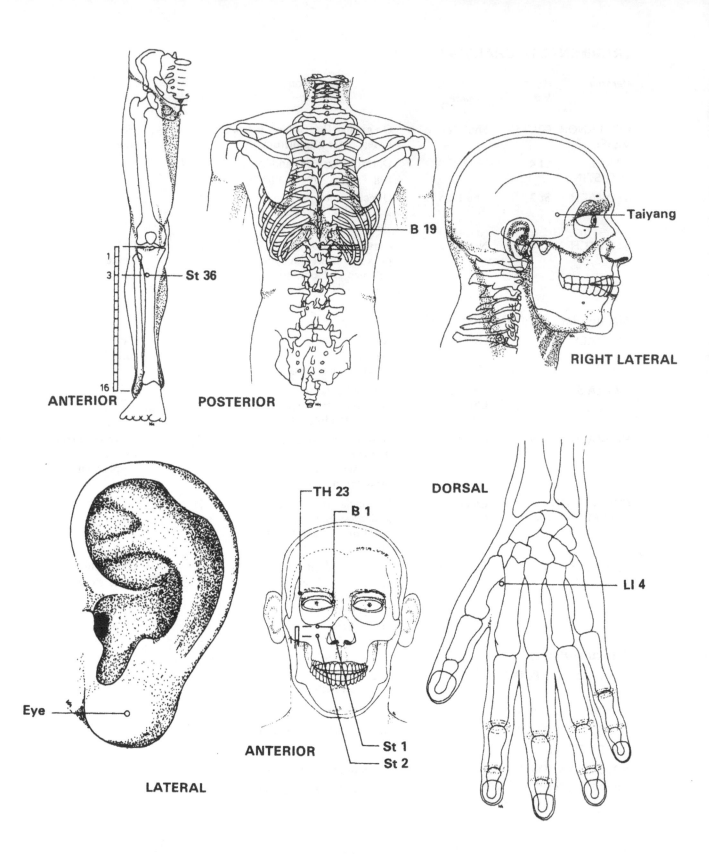

ANTERIOR

POSTERIOR

RIGHT LATERAL

B 19

St 36

Taiyang

TH 23

B 1

DORSAL

Eye

ANTERIOR

St 1
St 2

LI 4

LATERAL

114

EYE PAIN

The points in the immediate vicinity of the eye should be treated with the utmost caution regarding position and depth of insertion. Only mild stimulation should be given to these local points.

Conjunctivitis

Meridian	Point Ref	Chinese Name	Anatomical Position	Depth of Insertion (inches)	Special Note
BLADDER	B 1	Ching Ming	Just lateral and superior to inner canthus.	$\frac{1}{6}$	Insert needle very superficially with care. Do not rotate.
LARGE INTESTINE	LI 4	Ho Ku	Dorsal surface of hand in angle between 1st 2 metacarpals.	1	
EXTRA 2		Taiyang	In a depression 1 AUM posterior to midpoint between lateral end of eyebrow and outer canthus.	½ or 1	Perpendicularly or obliquely downwards
OR					
TRIPLE HEATER	TH 23	Ssŭ Chu K'ung	Lateral aspect of eyebrow.	¾	Horizontally posteriorly
STOMACH	St 1	Ch'eng Ch'i	Vertically below pupil, just below inferior edge of orbit.	$\frac{1}{6}$	Patient looking upwards as needle inserted perpendicularly.

Auricular Point

EYE POINT — Centre of ear-lobe.

Neuralgia Involving the Eye

Meridian	Point Ref	Chinese Name	Anatomical Position	Depth of Insertion (inches)	Special Note
BLADDER	B 19	Tan Yü	1½ AUM lateral to lower border of spinous process of 10th thoracic vertebra.	¼	
STOMACH	St 2	Ssŭ Pai	¾ AUM below Ch'eng Chi (see above)	¼ or 1	Perpendicularly or horizontally downwards.

For all eye conditions involving pain, add:

Meridian	Point Ref	Chinese Name	Anatomical Position	Depth of Insertion (inches)	Special Note
STOMACH	St 36	(Tsu) San Li	3 AUM inferior to knee crease, 1 finger's width lateral to crest of tibia	1	

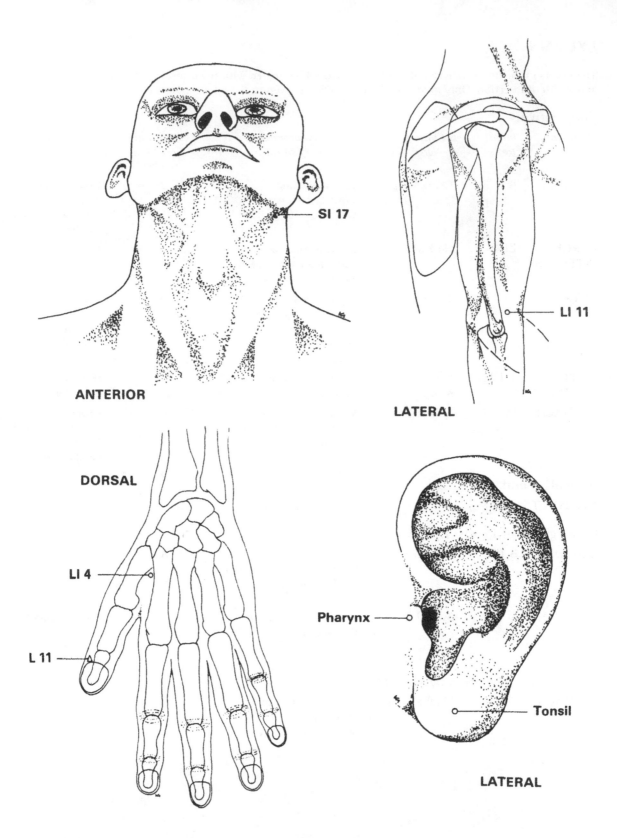

ANTERIOR

SI 17

LATERAL

LI 11

DORSAL

LI 4

L 11

Pharynx

Tonsil

LATERAL

THROAT PAIN

Suitable for such conditions as tonsillitis, pharyngitis, etc.

Meridian	Point Ref	Chinese Name	Anatomical Position	Depth of Insertion (inches)	Special Note
SMALL INTESTINE	SI 17	T'ien Yung	Immediately inferior and posterior to angle of jaw. On anterior border of sterno-cleidomastoid muscle.	1	
LARGE INTESTINE	LI 4	Ho Ku	Dorsal surface of hand in angle between 1st 2 metacarpals.	1	
LUNG	L 11	Shao Shang	Radial aspect of thumb just posterior to nail root.	$\frac{1}{10}$	Obliquely upwards. Cauterization forbidden.
LARGE INTESTINE	LI 11	Ch'ü Ch'ih	Lateral end of elbow crease. Between lateral epicondyle and edge of elbow fold.	1	

Auricular Points

PHARYNX POINT — Opposite external meatus on medial and superior aspect of tragus.

TONSIL POINT — Central lower aspect of ear-lobe.

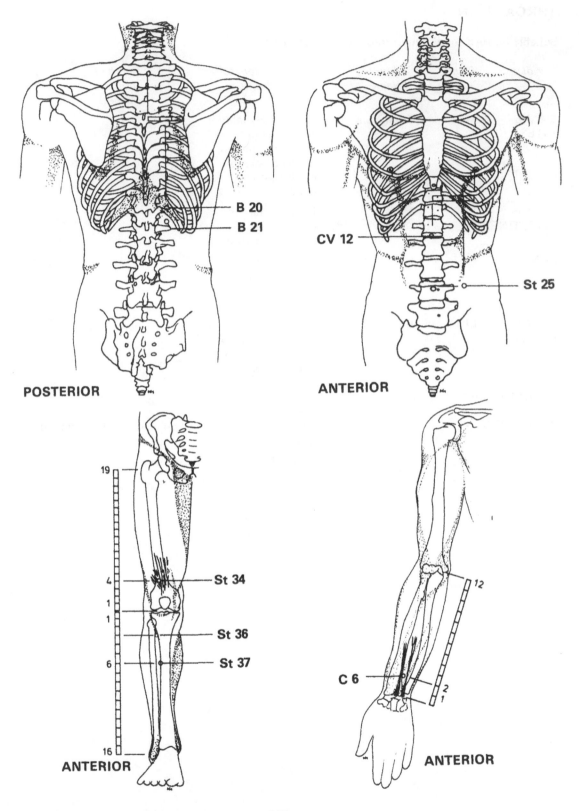

POSTERIOR

B 20
B 21

ANTERIOR

CV 12

St 25

19

4

1

1

St 34

St 36

St 37

6

16

ANTERIOR

12

C 6

2

1

ANTERIOR

118

ABDOMINAL PAIN

These points have a general regulating effect as well as diminishing abdominal pain and discomfort. In treatment of peptic ulcer it was found that points Stomach 36, (Tsu) San li, and Conception Vessel 12, Chung Kuan, not only suppressed pain but diminished the volume of gastric secretion and lowered the level of pepsin.[1]

Gastrointestinal Conditions

Meridian	Point Ref	Chinese Name	Anatomical Position	Depth of Insertion (inches)	Special Note
STOMACH	St 36	(Tsu) San Li	3 AUM inferior to knee crease, 1 finger's width lateral to crest of tibia.	1	
CONCEPTION VESSEL	CV 12	Chung Kuan	Midpoint between xyphoid process and umbilicus.	1	

Use strong stimulation leaving needle *in situ* 30-60 minutes; repeat stimulation manually every 10-15 minutes or use electrostimulation. Do not use cauterization during acute attacks. If pain is accompanied by nausea and vomiting, add:

Meridian	Point Ref	Chinese Name	Anatomical Position	Depth of Insertion (inches)	Special Note
CIRCULATION	C 6	Nei Kuan	Anterior surface of forearm 2 AUM proximal to wrist crease between radius and ulna.	¾	
STOMACH	St 25	T'ien Ch'u	3 AUM lateral to umbilicus.	¾	
STOMACH	St 37	(Tsu) Shang Lien[2]	Anterior surface of leg, 6 AUM inferior to knee crease, between tibia and fibula.	1	

If pain is acute, add:

Meridian	Point Ref	Chinese Name	Anatomical Position	Depth of Insertion (inches)	Special Note
STOMACH	St 34	Lian Ch' iu	Anterior surface of thigh between rectus femoris and vastus lateralis, 2 AUM superior to upper margin of patella.	1	

Other useful points are:

Meridian	Point Ref	Chinese Name	Anatomical Position	Depth of Insertion (inches)	Special Note
BLADDER	B 21	Wei Yü	1½ AUM lateral to inferior margin of 12th thoracic vertebra.	½	
BLADDER	B 20	P' i Yü	1½ AUM lateral to inferior margin of 11th thoracic vertebra.	½	

[1] *Chinese Medical Journal*, Vol. 1, No. 4, page 253, July 1975.
[2] Modern Chinese texts name this point Shang Chü Hsü.

continued overleaf

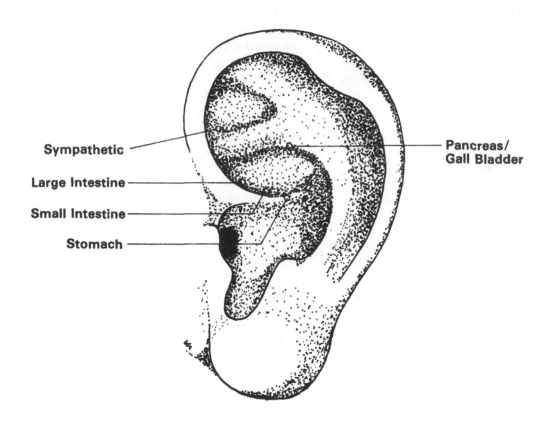

Sympathetic

Large Intestine

Small Intestine

Stomach

Pancreas/
Gall Bladder

LATERAL

120

ABDOMINAL PAIN (contd.)

Auricular Points

STOMACH POINT	Upper portion of helix crus.
SYMPATHETIC NERVE POINT	In deltoid fossa.
SMALL INTESTINE POINT	Centre of superior aspect of helix crus.
LARGE INTESTINE POINT	Antero-superior portion helix crus.
PANCREAS-GALL BLADDER POINT	Posterior portion of infra-antihelix crus.

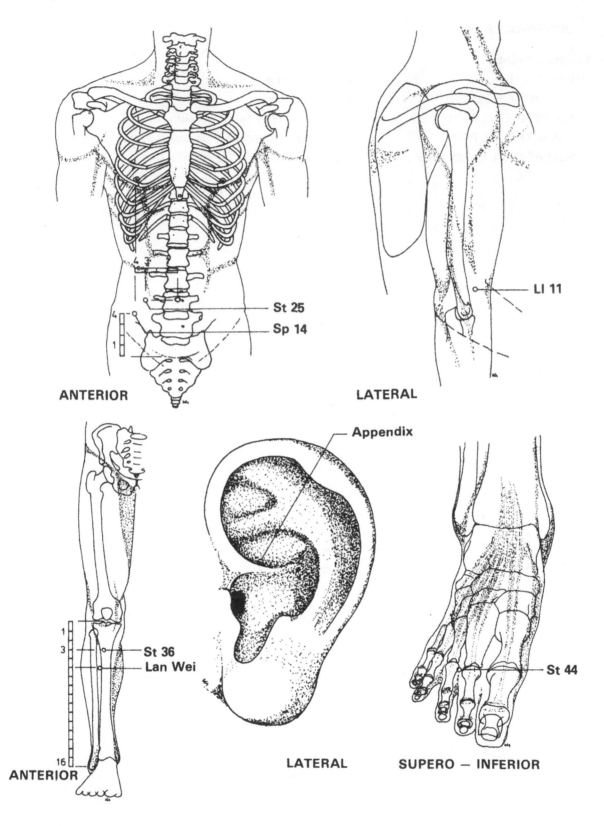

ANTERIOR

LATERAL

St 25

Sp 14

LI 11

ANTERIOR

St 36

Lan Wei

Appendix

LATERAL

SUPERO — INFERIOR

St 44

APPENDIX PAIN

Treat several times daily in acute condition. Needle should be left *in situ* for up to an hour and should be strongly manipulated every 10-15 minutes. It is not suggested that this is the only or the best way of treating acute appendictis, but as a component part of any other suitable form of treatment (fasting, medication, surgery, etc) it is invaluable.

Meridian	Point Ref	Chinese Name	Anatomical Position	Depth of Insertion (inches)	Special Note
STOMACH	St 36	(Tsu) San Li	3 AUM inferior to knee crease 1 finger's width lateral to crest of tibia.	1	
SPLEEN	Sp 14	Fu Chieh	4 AUM lateral to abdominal midline and 4 AUM above groin crease.	¾	
STOMACH	St 25	T'ien Ch'u	3 AUM lateral to umbilicus.	¾	
LARGE INTESTINE	LI 11	Ch'ü Ch'ih	At external aspect of elbow crease with elbow flexed. Between lateral epicondyle and edge of elbow fold.	1¼	
EXTRA 33		Lan Wei	5 AUM distal to knee crease on anterior surface of leg. Between tibia and fibula. The point will be sensitive to pressure in appendicitis.	1½	
STOMACH	St 44	Nei T'ing	Dorsal aspect of foot ½ AUM proximal to web margin between 2nd and 3rd metatarsals.	½	Obliquely upwards.

Auricular Point

APPENDIX POINT   Between centre and medial aspect of superior helix crus.

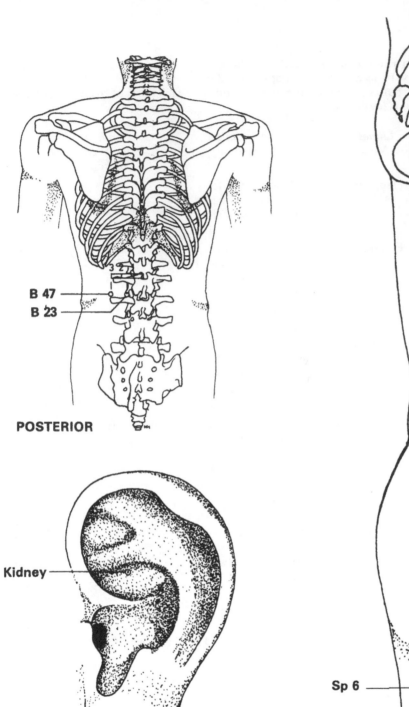

POSTERIOR

B 47
B 23

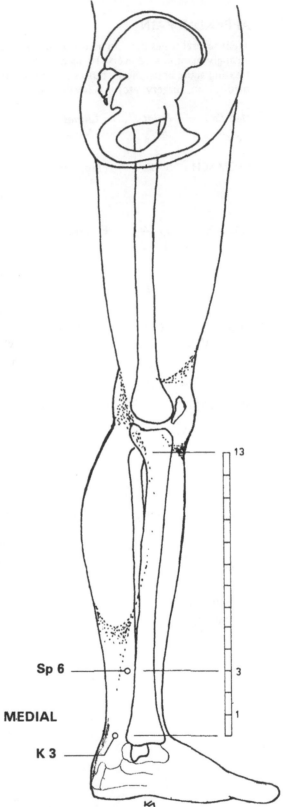

13

Sp 6

MEDIAL

K 3

3

1

Kidney

LATERAL

124

RENAL COLIC

Meridian	Point Ref	Chinese Name	Anatomical Position	Depth of Insertion (inches)	Special Note
BLADDER	B 23	Shen Yü	1½ AUM lateral to spine at level of interspace between 2nd and 3rd lumbar vertebrae.	¾	
SPLEEN	Sp 6	San Yin Chiao	3 AUM[1] proximal to medial malleolus, just posterior to tibia.	1	
BLADDER	B 47	Chih Shih	3 AUM lateral to spine at level of interspace between 2nd and 3rd lumbar vertebrae.	½ or 1½	Perpendicularly or obliquely caudad or cephalid.
KIDNEY	K 3	T'ai Ch'i	At level of medial malleolus midway between its posterior border and Achilles tendon.	½	

Auricular Point

KIDNEY POINT — At lower border of infra-antihelix crus.

---

[1] Note some Western authorities give this as 4 AUM.

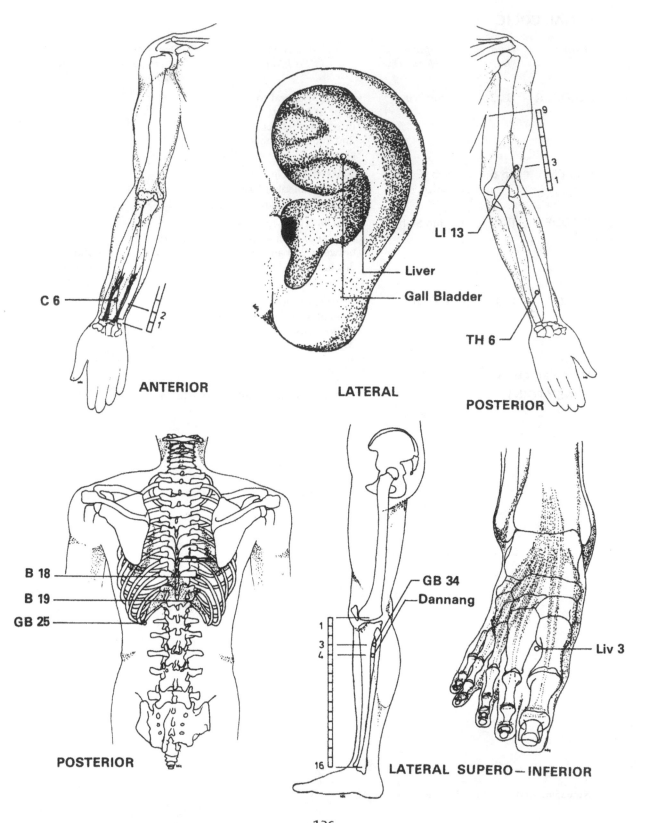

ANTERIOR

C 6

2
1

LATERAL

Liver

Gall Bladder

POSTERIOR

LI 13

TH 6

9
3
1

POSTERIOR

B 18
B 19
GB 25

LATERAL SUPERO—INFERIOR

GB 34
Dannang

1
3
4

16

Liv 3

126

BILIARY COLIC

Meridian	Point Ref	Chinese Name	Anatomical Position	Depth of Insertion (inches)	Special Note
Extra 35		Dannang	Approximately 1½ AUM distal to depression anterior to head of fibula. Tender on digital pressure in cases of gall bladder or bile-duct dysfunction.	1	
CIRCULATION	C 6	Nei Kuan	2 AUM proximal to wrist crease between tendons of flexor carpi radialis and palmaris longus.	¾	

The following points may be added, but on the right side only.

Meridian	Point Ref	Chinese Name	Anatomical Position	Depth of Insertion (inches)	Special Note
LARGE INTESTINE	LI 13	(Yang) Wu Li	Antero-medial border of humerus. 3 AUM proximal to elbow crease.	1	Take care to avoid artery . Insert perpendicularly.
GALL BLADDER	GB 25	Ching Men	At lower border of free end of 12th rib.	$\frac{1}{3}$	

Auricular Points

GALL BLADDER POINT		Posterior portion of infra-antihelix crus.
LIVER POINT		Posterior border of concha level of helix crus.

The following points may be helpful if the above fail to relieve pain.

Meridian	Point Ref	Chinese Name	Anatomical Position	Depth of Insertion (inches)	Special Note
BLADDER	B 18	Kan Yü	1½ AUM lateral to lower border of spinous process of 9th thoracic vertebrae.	½	
BLADDER	B 19	Tan Yü	1½ AUM lateral to lower border of spinous process of 10th thoracic vertebrae.	½	
GALL BLADDER	GB 34	Yang Ling Ch'üan	3 AUM below knee crease in a depression anterior and inferior to head of fibula.	1–1½	
LIVER	Liv 3	T'ai Ch'ung	Between 1st and 2nd toe, 2 AUM proximal to web margin.	¾	Obliquely upwards.
TRIPLE HEATER	TH 6	Chih Kou	3 AUM proximal to dorsal wrist crease between radius and ulna.	¾	

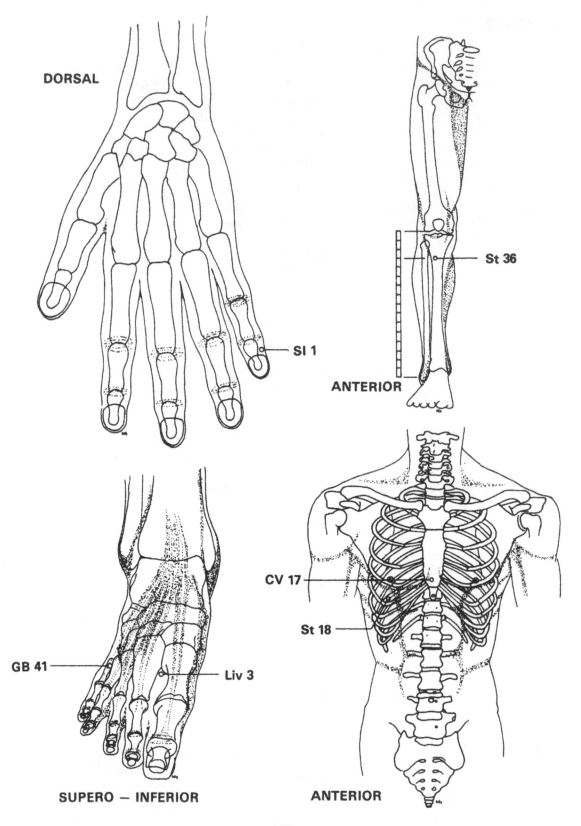

DORSAL

SI 1

St 36

ANTERIOR

GB 41

Liv 3

CV 17

St 18

SUPERO — INFERIOR

ANTERIOR

128

BREAST PAIN

Select 2 or 3 of the following for each treatment.

Meridian	Point Ref	Chinese Name	Anatomical Position	Depth of Insertion (inches)	Special Note
LIVER	Liv 3	T'ai Ch'ung	Between 1st and 2nd toe, 2 AUM proximal to web margin.	¾	
STOMACH	St 18	Ju Ken	In 5th intercostal space below the nipple.	¾	Obliquely.
STOMACH	St 36	(Tsu) San Li	3 AUM distal to knee crease, 1 finger's width lateral to anterior crest of tibia.	1¼	
CONCEPTION VESSEL	CV 17	Hsien Chung	At the point midway between nipples (patient supine).	¾	Angle needle laterally or downwards.
SMALL INTESTINE	SI 1	Shao Chih	$\frac{1}{10}$ AUM proximal to external corner of little finger nail.	$\frac{1}{10}$	
GALL BLADDER	GB 41	(Tsu) Lin Ch'i	In depression anterior to junction of 4th and 5th metatarsals.	¾	

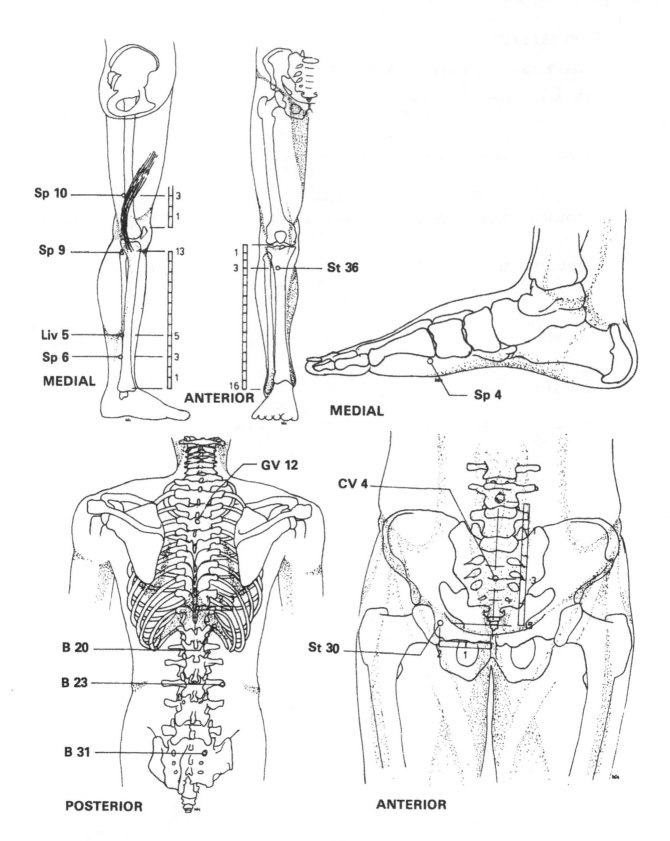

Sp 10

Sp 9

Liv 5

Sp 6

MEDIAL

3

1

13

5

3

1

ANTERIOR

1

3

16

St 36

MEDIAL

Sp 4

GV 12

CV 4

B 20

B 23

B 31

St 30

POSTERIOR

ANTERIOR

130

MENSTRUAL PAIN

Meridian	Point Ref	Chinese Name	Anatomical Position	Depth of Insertion (inches)	Special Note
CONCEPTION VESSEL	CV 4	Kuan Yuan	3 AUM inferior to umbilicus.	1¼	
SPLEEN	Sp 6	San Yin Chiao	3 AUM[1] above tip of internal malleolus, just posterior to tibial border.	1	

For pelvic inflammation:

STOMACH	St 30	Ch'i Ch'ung	5 AUM inferior to umbilicus and 2 AUM lateral to midline.	¾	
LIVER	Liv 5	Li Kou	5 AUM superior to medial malleolus, on posterior border of tibia.	1	

For menstrual irregularity:

SPLEEN	Sp 10	Hsüeh Hai	2 AUM proximal to superior border of patella on antero-medial surface of thigh, just posterior to sartorious.	1	
STOMACH	St 36	(Tsu) San Li	3 AUM inferior to knee crease 1 finger's width lateral to crest of tibia.	1¼	
SPLEEN	Sp 9	Yin Ling Ch'üan	Level with medial prominence of tibia, in a depression on lower border of condyle.	1	Cauterization forbidden.
BLADDER	B 20	P'i Yü	1½ AUM lateral to lower border of 11th thoracic spinous process.	½	

For menstrual cramp:

SPLEEN	Sp 4	Kung Sun	Medial aspect of foot in a depression at anterior, inferior border of 1st metatarsal.	¾	

[1] Note some Western authorities give this as 4 AUM.

continued overleaf

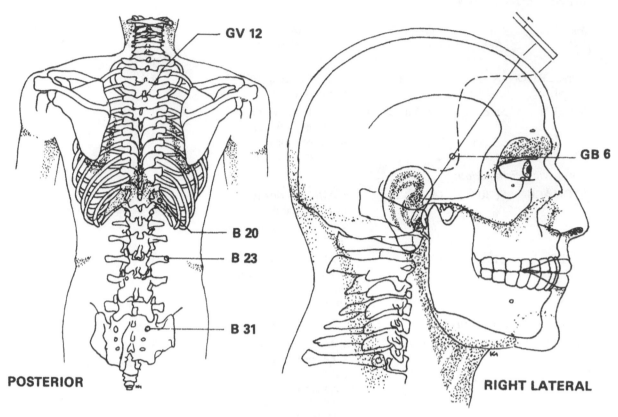

GV 12

B 20

B 23

B 31

POSTERIOR

GB 6

RIGHT LATERAL

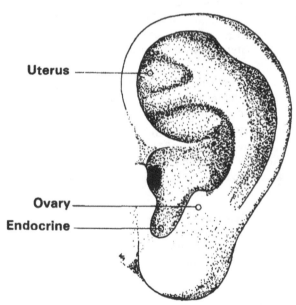

Uterus

Ovary

Endocrine

LATERAL

MENSTRUAL PAIN (contd.)

Meridian	Point Ref	Chinese Name	Anatomical Position	Depth of Insertion (inches)	Special Note
Other useful points are:					
GOVERNOR VESSEL	GV 12	Shen Chu	Immediately inferior to spinous process of 3rd thoracic vertebra.	¾	Insert needle obliquely upwards.
BLADDER	B 23	Shen Yü	1½ AUM lateral to lower border of 2nd lumbar spinous process.	1	
BLADDER	B 31	Shang Liao	In 1st sacral foramen.	1	
GALL BLADDER	GB 6	Hsüan Li	On line connecting external auditory meatus and a point on midline ½ AUM above anterior hairline. This point is 1 AUM inferior to midpoint of this line.	¼	

Auricular Points

UTERUS POINT	In middle of border of deltoid fossa of helix.
OVARY POINT	On lower aspect of interior wall of antitragus.
ENDOCRINE POINT	Inferior to tragic notch on cavum conchae.

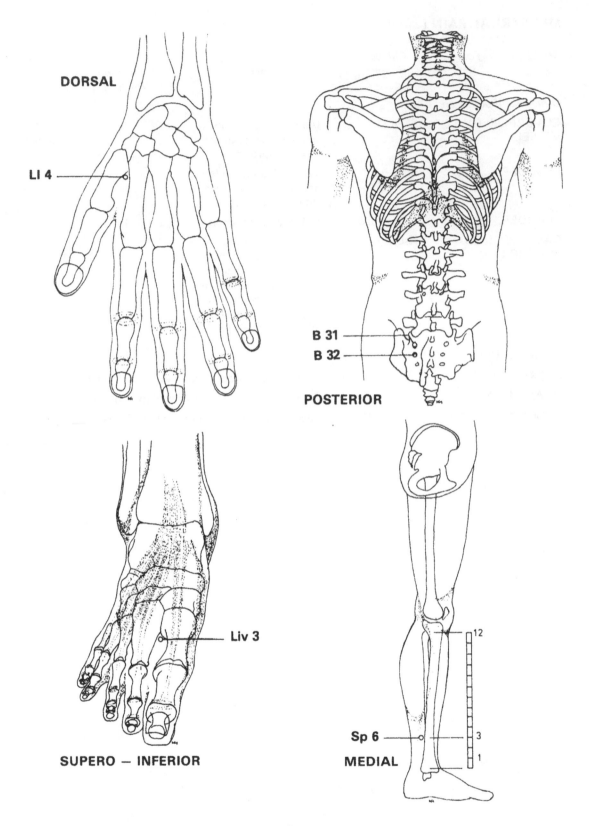

DORSAL

LI 4

POSTERIOR

B 31
B 32

SUPERO — INFERIOR

Liv 3

MEDIAL

Sp 6

12

3

1

LABOUR PAIN

The following points will reduce pain and facilitate delivery.

Meridian	Point Ref	Chinese Name	Anatomical Position	Depth of Insertion (inches)	Special Note
SPLEEN	Sp 6	San Yin Chiao	3 AUM[1] proximal to medial malleolus, just posterior to tibia.	1	
LIVER	Liv 3	T'ai Ch'ung	Between 1st and 2nd toes, 2 AUM proximal to web margin.	¾	
BLADDER	B 31	Shang Liao	In 1st sacral foramen.	1	
BLADDER	B 32	Tz'ŭ Liao	In 2nd sacral foramen.	1	
LARGE INTESTINE	LI 4	Ho Ku	Dorsal surface of hand in angle of 1st 2 metacarpals.	1	

All points should be strongly stimulated for up to 30 minutes.

[1] Note some Western authorities give this as 4 AUM.

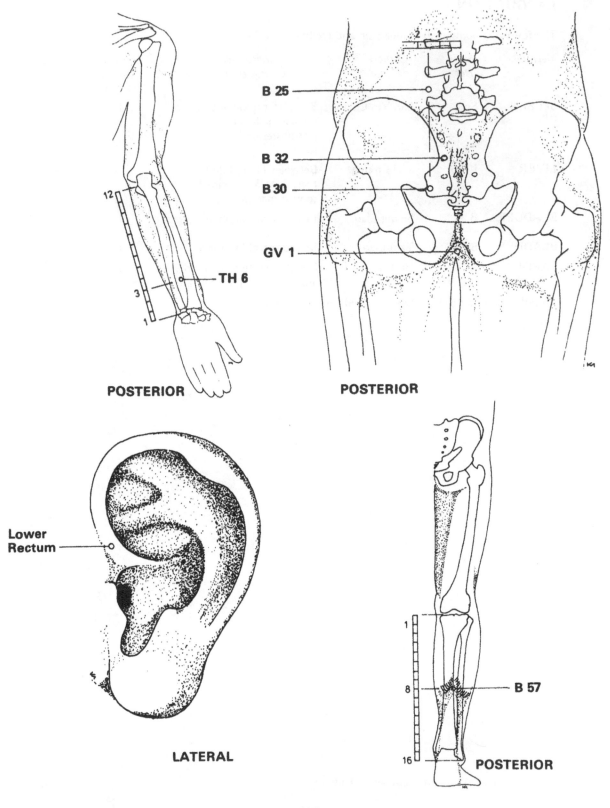

POSTERIOR

B 25
B 32
B 30
GV 1

POSTERIOR

TH 6

Lower
Rectum

LATERAL

B 57

POSTERIOR

136

ANAL PAIN (Haemorrhoids).

Meridian	Point Ref	Chinese Name	Anatomical Position	Depth of Insertion (inches)	Special Note
BLADDER	B 25	T'a Ch'ang Yü	1½ AUM lateral to lower aspect of spinous process of 4th lumbar vertebra.	1	
BLADDER	B 30	Pai Huan Yü	1½ AUM lateral to midline in level of 4th sacral foramen.	1	
BLADDER	B 32	Tz'ŏ Liao	In 2nd sacral foramen.	1	
BLADDER	B 57	Ch'eng Shan	8 AUM below knee crease inferior to belly of gastrocnemius.	1¼	
GOVERNOR VESSEL	GV 1	Ch'ang Ch'iang	Midway between tip of coccyx and anus.	¾	
TRIPLE HEATER	TH 6	Chih Kou	Posterior surface of forearm between radius and ulna, 3 AUM proximal to wrist crease.	¾	

Auricular Points

LOWER RECTUM POINT   On helix, directly superior to external meatus.

137

Acupuncture Anaesthesia

Acupuncture analgesia is a better description of this phenomenon. The Greek word *anaisthësia* means 'lack of sensation'. In acupuncture anaesthesia the only sensation that is diminished is that of pain. Analgesia literally means insensibility to pain without loss of consciousness. However, the semantics of the phenomenon are relatively unimportant when compared with its enormous potential.

The technique is safe. It allows the patient to remain fully conscious during surgery. The patient's physiological functions remain relatively stable throughout surgery and post-operative recovery is enhanced. The use of this method of anaesthesia is obviously indicated in seriously ill or debilitated patients. In brain surgery, for example, it is an advantage to the surgeon to have a patient who is able to respond to instructions or questions throughout the period of surgery.

It is essential that the patient is mentally prepared for this form of anaesthetic. He must be calm and relaxed, and each stage of the surgical procedure must be explained so that he does not panic. The sensations of stretching which occur in abdominal surgery, for example, will require a degree of fortitude on the part of the patient. It may be that acupuncture anaesthesia will not be entirely suitable for abdominal surgery until the technique has been completely perfected. Certainly where is is anticipated that visceral traction will be marked, other techniques of anaesthesia would be preferable. Analgesia is more successful in thoracic, neck and head surgery. If the patient is obviously nervous, sceptical or apprehensive, however, it may be undesirable to press on with acupuncture anaesthesia at all.

In all cases a needling test should be carried out prior to surgery. This is to assess the patient's sensitivity and tolerance to acupuncture. At this time the operative procedure should be described in order to prepare the patient and to calm anxieties.

The means whereby points have been selected differ. In some cases points on meridians that traverse the operation site or relate directly to the organ involved are selected. This method, together with clinical experience of body and auricular points, has led to a gradual perfection of technique. At one time many points were stimulated in order to anaesthetize the patient; refinement of techniques has, however, led to many surgical procedures being possible with only one point of stimulation.

The technique is similar to normal body or auricular acupuncture. Depth of insertion will vary according to the patient's body type, though one and a half to three centimetres is usual.

Insertion should be swift and should be followed by rotation combined with lifting and thrusting of the needle. The degree of rotation is between ninety and 360 degrees. The range of the lifting and thrusting of the needle is from 0.5 to one centimetre, and this is performed by the index and middle fingers, whilst the rotation is achieved by the thumb. The speed of movement is between 100 and 200 times per minute. The induction time from needling to the first incision takes fifteen to thirty minutes. The technique requires a smooth, even use of the needle. The angle of the needle's insertion should remain the same throughout the procedure. The degree of stimulation must always be tolerable to the patient, who should be able to describe a feeling of soreness, distension and heaviness.

The needle may be connected to an electric pulse stimulator. The outputs most commonly used in China are in the form of biphasic spike waves, biphasic square waves or sinusoidal waves. The frequency may range from twenty per minute to several hundred per second. Starting with a low frequency, the intensity is gradually increased until the patient reports a feeling of numbness and distension. The local musculature should quiver slightly and the patient should report a degree of local irritation. After a short while, these sensations may decrease and the electrical stimulation should be increased to maintain the subjective sensations and the muscular quiver.

It should be realized that, whilst ostensibly similar, the electrical stimulation of acupuncture needles, in situ, is not the same procedure as trans-cutaneous nerve stimulation. This latter method is performed with electrodes which do not pierce the skin and is also primarily aimed at stimulating neural structures, which is not necessarily the aim of acupuncture. Both these methods do, however, appear to stimulate the production of endogenous polypeptides (endorphins). As a rule the power supply (battery, or mains via transformer) is between 3 and 6 volts with output of between 25 and 200 microamperes.

To achieve the analgesic/anaesthetic effect the use of pulsating waves, with a saw-tooth wave, is the most effective. For this purpose square and sine waves are ineffective and might prove painful.

A variety of physiological effects result from electro-acupuncture, and to a large extent these are dependent on the choice of points, the type, strength and length of the stimulation imparted. It is worth repeating that the subjective sensation should be of heaviness, paresthesia, perhaps mild aching, but no pain.

If the point of insertion should bleed or if the desired sensations are not felt by the patient, the needle should be removed and a new point selected. The needle should never be inserted all the way to its handle in case it fractures.

Certain pre- and post-operative adjuvant drugs are used in China in exceptional circumstances. The Chinese surgeons use such measures during, for example, the separation of the periostium or traction of internal organs, and also if the patient becomes restless or apprehensive. However, in the vast majority of the hundreds of thousands of surgical procedures using acupuncture anaesthesia peformed in China in recent years, no additional medication has been required.

The degree of effectiveness in certain types of operations is as follows[1]

Craniotomy	606 cases	96.2%	effective surgery with acupuncture anaesthesia used.
Thyroid	670 cases	95.4%	effective

[1]*Chinese Medical Journal,* Vol. 1, No 1, January, 1975.

Detached Retina	1374 cases	80.7%	effective
Pulmonary Resection	656 cases	96.5%	effective
Subtotal Gastrectomy	763 cases	96.1%	effective
Abdominal Hysterectomy	590 cases	87.4%	effective
Internal fixation of fracture with three-flanged nail.	462 cases	96.5%	effective

The Shanghai Acupuncture Anaesthesia Co-ordinating Group, who compiled the report mentioned above, remark that pain abatement is incomplete under acupuncture anaesthesia, and that some patients feel varying degrees of pain. A further clinical problem is that muscle relaxation is not fully adequate, especially in abdominal surgery. In thoracic surgery the patient is instructed in abdominal breathing but patients should nevertheless anticipate some unpleasant sensations.

The advantages, however, far outweigh the relatively few, as yet unsolved problems. For example, in a series of 100 mitral commissurotomies performed under acupuncture anaesthesia, the patient's blood-pressure remained perfectly stable throughout.

The recovery stages in the majority of patients after surgery under acupuncture anaesthesia were uncomplicated and speedy. There were far fewer cases of post-operative infection, abdominal distension or urinary retention.

The points on the following pages are those recommended by the Academy of Traditional Chinese Medicine and the Shanghai Acupuncture Anaesthesia Co-ordinating Group.

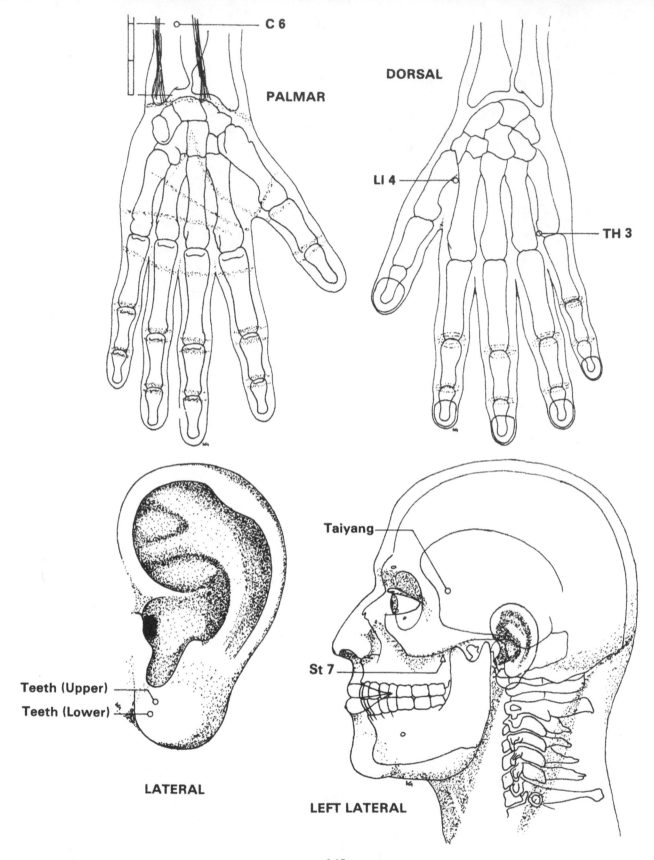

PALMAR

C 6

DORSAL

LI 4

TH 3

LATERAL

Teeth (Upper)

Teeth (Lower)

Taiyang

St 7

LEFT LATERAL

ANAESTHESIA FOR TONSILLECTOMY

Meridian	Point Ref	Chinese Name	Anatomical Position	Special Note
Prescription 1				
LARGE INTESTINE	LI 4	Ho Ku	Dorsal surface of hand in angle of 1st 2 meta-carpals.	Bilaterally.
Prescription 2				
LARGE INTESTINE and TRIPLE HEATER	LI 4 TH 3	Ho Ku Chung Chu	Dorsum of hand between 4th and 5th metacarpal bones in a depression posterior to metacarpo-phalangeal joint.	Stimulate electrically.
OR				
CIRCULATION	C6	Nei Kuan	2 AUM above wrist crease between tendons of palmaris longus and flexor carpi radialis.	

ANAESTHESIA FOR TOOTH EXTRACTION

Meridian	Point Ref	Chinese Name	Anatomical Position	Special Note
Prescription 1				
LARGE INTESTINE	LI 4	Ho Ku	Dorsal surface of hand in angle of 1st 2 meta-carpals.	Both sides or affected side.
Prescription 2				
EXTRA 2		Taiyang	In depression 1 AUM posterior to midpoint between lateral end of eyebrow and outer canthus.	Stimulate manually or electrically.
Penetrate towards:				
STOMACH	St 7	Hsia Kuan	In depression at lower border of zygomatic arch, anterior to condyle of mandible.	Cauterization forbidden.

Prescription 3

Auricular Points

Meridian	Point Ref	Chinese Name	Anatomical Position	Special Note
TEETH (UPPER) POINT *or* TEETH (LOWER) POINT				Stimulate electrically.

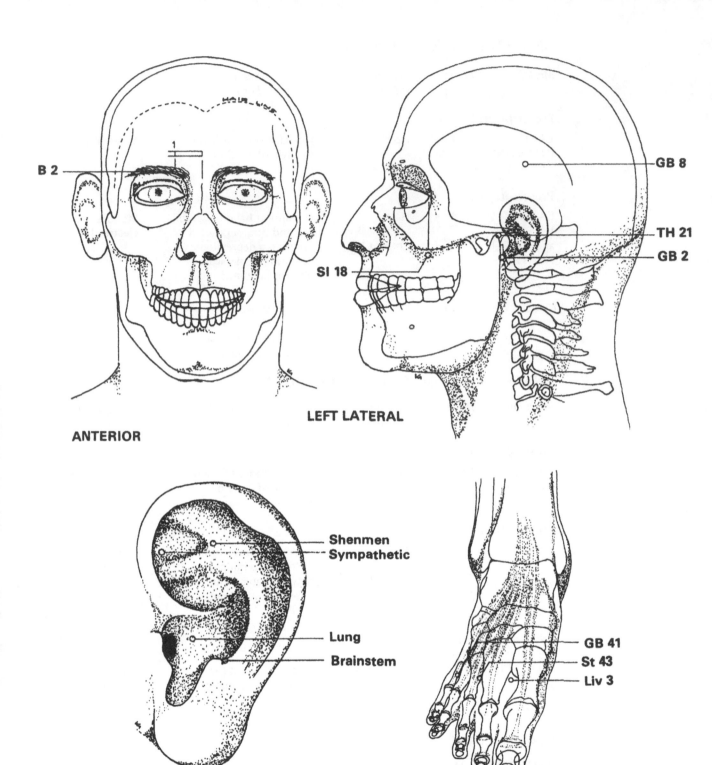

B 2

ANTERIOR

LEFT LATERAL

GB 8

TH 21

GB 2

SI 18

Shenmen
Sympathetic

Lung

Brainstem

LATERAL

GB 41
St 43
Liv 3

SUPERO — INFERIOR

ANAESTHESIA FOR CRANIAL SURGERY

Meridian	Point Ref	Chinese Name	Anatomical Position	Special Note
Prescription 1				
SMALL INTESTINE	SI 18	Ch'üan Liao	Directly below outer canthus in depression below lower border of zygomatic bone.	
LIVER	Liv 3	(T'ai) Ch'ung	Dorsal surface of foot at angle between 1st and 2nd metatarsals.	Stimulate electrically.
STOMACH	St 43	Hsien Ku	Dorsal surface of foot at angle between 2nd and 3rd metatarsals.	
GALL BLADDER	GB 41	(Tsu) Lin Ch'i	Dorsal surface of foot at angle between 4th and 5th metatarsals.	
Prescription 2				
TRIPLE HEATER	TH 21	Erh Men	Anterior to auricle at apex of angle formed by tragus and helix.	Stimulate electrically.
Penetrate towards:				
GALL BLADDER	GB 2	T'ing Hui	Anterior to ear-lobe, posterior to condyle of mandible.	
BLADDER	B 2	Ts'uan Chu	Extreme medial aspect of eyebrow 1 AUM from median line.	
GALL BLADDER	GB 8	Shuai Ku	If auricle is folded forward, this point is directly above apex.	

Prescription 3

Auricular Points

EAR SHENMEN POINT   Needle directed towards Kidney Point.

BRAINSTEM POINT   Needle towards Subcortex Point.

SYMPATHETIC NERVE POINT

LUNG POINT

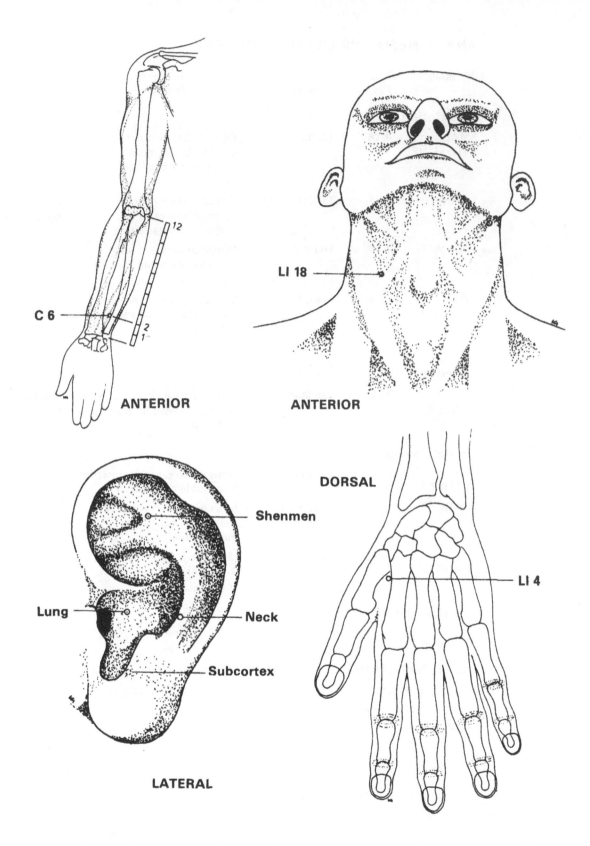

ANTERIOR

ANTERIOR

C 6

LI 18

12

2

1

DORSAL

Shenmen

Lung

Neck

Subcortex

LI 4

LATERAL

ANAESTHESIA FOR THYROID SURGERY

Meridian	Point Ref	Chinese Name	Anatomical Position	Special Note
Prescription 1				
LARGE INTESTINE	LI 4	Ho Ku	Dorsal surface of hand in angle of 1st 2 metacarpals.	Bilaterally *or* affected side only.
CIRCULATION	C6	Nei Kuan	On anterior surface of forearm between ulna and radius 2 AUM above wrist crease.	Stimulate electrically.
Prescription 2				
LARGE INTESTINE	LI 18	Fu Tu	3 AUM lateral to thyroid cartilage, between sternal head and clavicular head of sterno-cleido-mastoid muscle.	Bilaterally stimulate electrically.
Prescription 3				
Auricular Points				
EAR SHENMEN POINT			SUBCORTEX POINT	Stimulate
LUNG POINT		*OR*	NECK POINT	electrically.

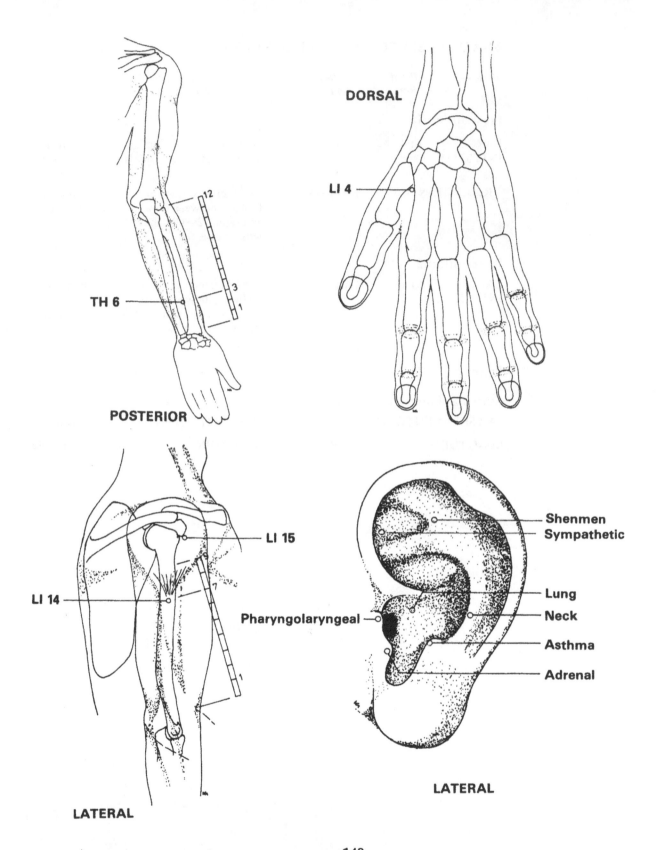

DORSAL

LI 4

TH 6

POSTERIOR

LI 15

LI 14

Pharyngolaryngeal

Shenmen
Sympathetic

Lung

Neck

Asthma

Adrenal

LATERAL

LATERAL

148

ANAESTHESIA FOR TOTAL LARYNGECTOMY

(Prescription of Eye, Ear, Nose and Throat Hospital of Shanghai First Medical College)

Meridian	Point Ref	Chinese Name	Anatomical Position	Special Note
Prescription 1				
LARGE INTESTINE	LI 4	Ho Ku	Dorsal surface of hand in angle of 1st 2 metacarpals.	Stimulate electrically left side only.
TRIPLE HEATER	TH 6	Chih Kou	On posterior arm surface, between uma and radius, 3 AUM above wrist.	

Prescription 2

Auricular Points

LUNG POINT

EAR SHENMEN POINT, needle directed towards Sympathetic Point.

ADRENAL GLAND POINT, needle directed towards Pharyngolaryngeal Point.

NECK POINT, needle directed towards Asthma Relieving point (Ding Chuan).

All electrically stimulated, bilaterally.

ANAESTHESIA FOR PULMONARY RESECTION

(Prescription of Shanghai First Tuberculosis Hospital)

Meridian	Point Ref	Chinese Name	Anatomical Position	Special Note
LARGE INTESTINE	LI 14	Pi Nao	Lateral surface of arm, at deltoid insertion. 7 AUM above elbow fold.	Hand stimulation on side of surgery.
Needle directed towards: LARGE INTESTINE	LI 15	Chien Mü	Anterior-inferior border of acromio-clavicular joint, inferior to acromion when arm is in abduction.	

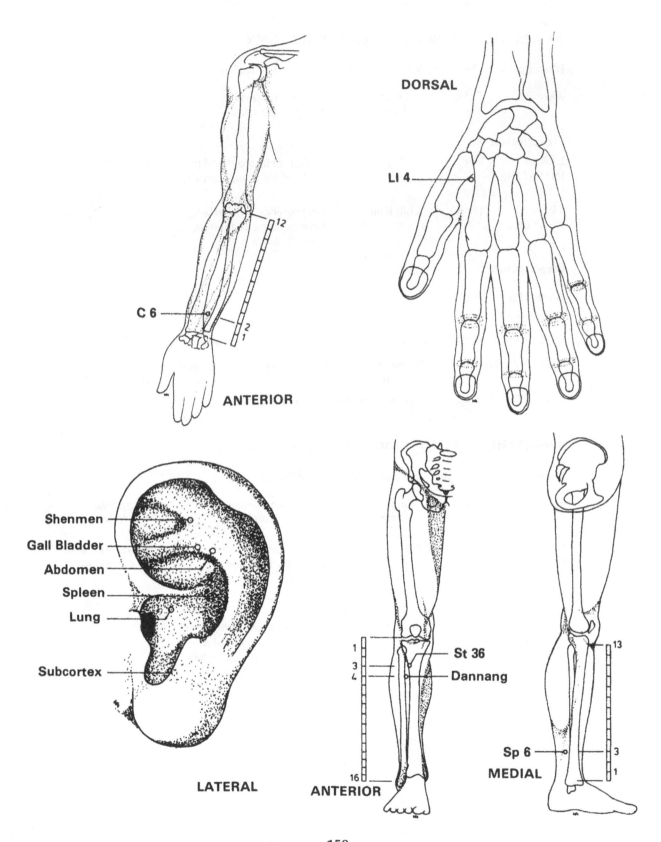

DORSAL

LI 4

ANTERIOR

C 6

12

2

1

Shenmen

Gall Bladder

Abdomen

Spleen

Lung

Subcortex

LATERAL

St 36

Dannang

ANTERIOR

1

3

4

16

Sp 6

MEDIAL

13

3

1

ANAESTHESIA FOR CHOLECYSTECTOMY AND SPLENECTOMY

Meridian	Point Ref	Chinese Name	Anatomical Position	Special Note
Prescription 1				
STOMACH	St 36	(Tsu) San Li	Antero-lateral aspect of leg 3 AUM below knee crease, 1 finger's width lateral to crest of tibia.	Bilaterally.
SPLEEN	Sp 6	San Yin Chiao	3 AUM[1] above tip of medial malleolus, just posterior to tibial border.	
EXTRA 35		Dannang	4 AUM below the knee crease about 1 AUM inferior and interior to small head of fibula. Sensitive to pressure.	
Prescription 2				
STOMACH	St 36	(Tsu) San Li	Antero-lateral aspect of leg 3 AUM below knee crease, 1 finger's width lateral to crest of tibia.	Bilaterally.
LARGE INTESTINE	LI 4	Ho Ku	Dorsal surface of hand in angle between 1st 2 metacarpals.	Bilaterally.
CIRCULATION	C6	Nei Kuan	2 AUM above wrist crease between tendons of palmaris longus and flexor carpi radialis.	Bilaterally.

Prescription 3

Auricular Points

GALL BLADDER POINT				Electric stimulation.
SPLEEN POINT				
ABDOMEN POINT				
EAR SHENMEN POINT				Bilaterally.
LUNG POINT				
SUBCORTEX POINT				

[1] Note some Western authorities give this as 4 AUM.

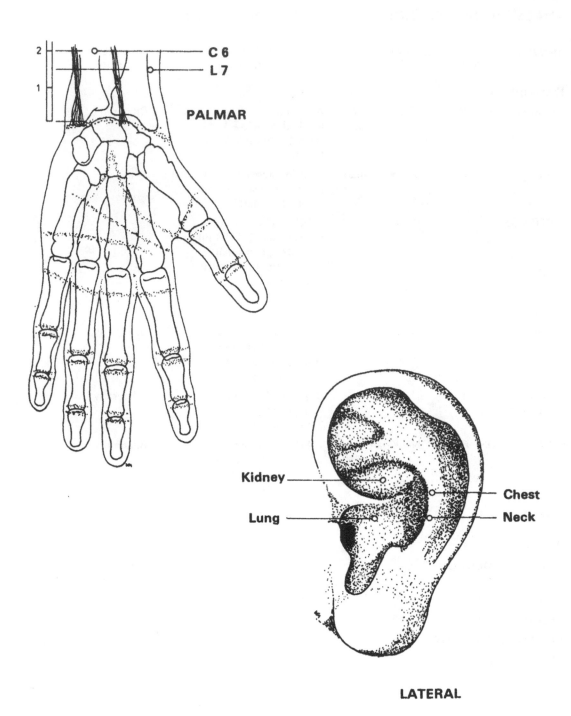

2
C 6
L 7
1

PALMAR

Kidney

Lung

Chest

Neck

LATERAL

152

ANAESTHESIA FOR OPEN HEART SURGERY

(Prescription of Third People's Hospital of Shanghai Second Medical College)

Meridian	Point Ref	Chinese Name	Anatomical Position	Special Note
LUNG	L 7	Lieh Ch'üeh	1½ AUM above distal wrist crease, above styloid process of radius.	Insertion obliquely upwards.
CIRCULATION	C6	Nei Kuan	Anterior surface of forearm between ulna and radius 2 AUM above wrist crease.	Stimulate both electrically, bilaterally.

OR

Auricular Points

NECK POINT
CHEST POINT
LUNG POINT
KIDNEY POINT

Left side only, stimulated electrically.

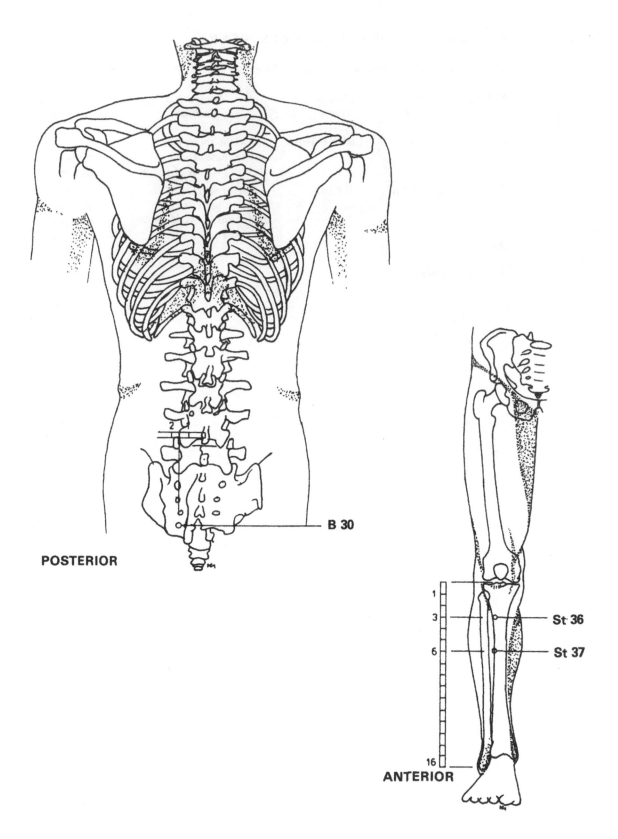

POSTERIOR

B 30

ANTERIOR

St 36

St 37

154

ANAESTHESIA FOR SURGERY TO LIGATE HAEMORRHOIDS

Meridian	Point Ref	Chinese Name	Anatomical Position	Special Note
BLADDER	B 30	Pai Huan Yü	At level of 4th sacral foramen, 1½ AUM lateral to midline.	Electrical stimulation, bilaterally.

ANAESTHESIA FOR SUBTOTAL GASTRECTOMY

Meridian	Point Ref	Chinese Name	Anatomical Position	Special Note
STOMACH	St 36	(Tsu) San Li	Antero-lateral aspect of leg, 3 AUM below knee crease, 1 finger's width lateral to crest of tibia.	Bilaterally.
STOMACH	St 37	(Tsu) Shang Lien[1]	Antero-lateral aspect of leg 6 AUM below knee crease, 1 finger's width lateral to crest of tibia.	Mechanically stimulated.

[1] Modern Chinese texts name this point Shang Chü Hsü.

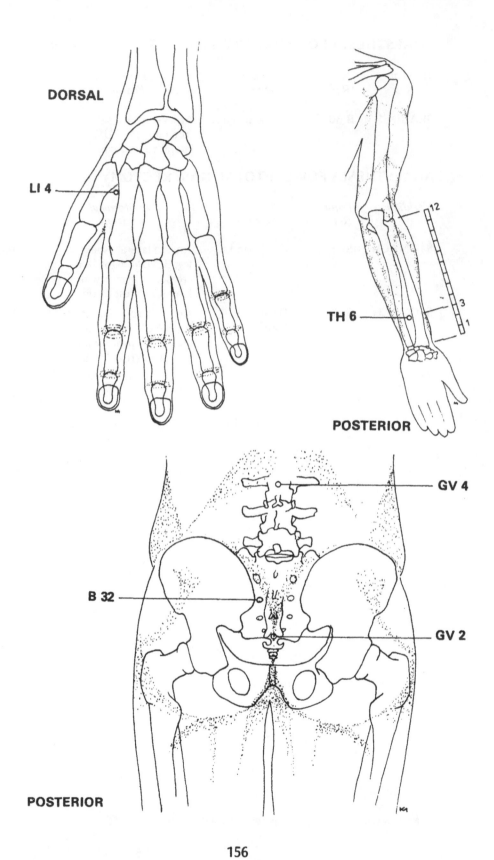

DORSAL

LI 4

TH 6

POSTERIOR

GV 4

B 32

GV 2

POSTERIOR

156

ANAESTHESIA FOR SURGERY TO REPAIR DETACHED RETINA

(Prescription of Shanghai First People's Hospital)

Meridian	Point Ref	Chinese Name	Anatomical Position	Special Note
LARGE INTESTINE	LI 4	Ho Ku	Dorsal surface of hand in angle of 1st 2 metacarpals.	Hand stimulation on side of surgery.
TRIPLE HEATER	TH 6	Chih Kou	3 AUM above wrist crease on posterior aspect of arm, between radius and ulna.	

ANAESTHESIA FOR ABDOMINAL HYSTERECTOMY

Meridian	Point Ref	Chinese Name	Anatomical Position	Special Note
BLADDER	B 32	Tz'ǔ Liao	On 2nd sacral foramen midway between median line and inferior aspect of postero-superior iliac crest.	Bilaterally.
GOVERNOR VESSEL	GV 2	Yao Yü	Junction of sacrum and coccyx at sacral hiatus.	Electrical stimulation.
GOVERNOR VESSEL	GV 4	Ming Men	Between 2nd and 3rd lumbar spinous processes.	

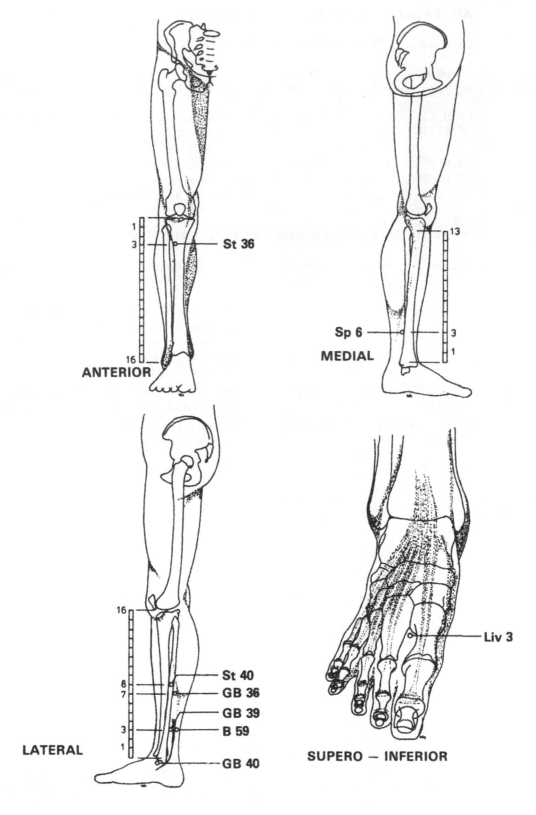

ANTERIOR

St 36

MEDIAL

Sp 6

13

3

1

LATERAL

16

St 40

GB 36

GB 39

B 59

GB 40

8

7

3

1

SUPERO — INFERIOR

Liv 3

158

ANAESTHESIA FOR SURGERY FOR FIXATION OF FRACTURE OF NECK OF FEMUR

Meridian	Point Ref	Chinese Name	Anatomical Position	Special Note
Prescription 1				
STOMACH	St 36	(Tsu) San Li	Antero-lateral aspect of leg, 3 AUM below knee crease, 1 finger's width lateral to crest of tibia.	All on
LIVER	Liv 3	T'ai Ch'ung	The depression between 1st and 2nd metatarsals, 2 AUM proximal to web.	the
GALL BLADDER	GB 40	Ch'iu Ch'ü	Anterior and inferior to external malleolus in depression lateral to tendon of extensor digitorum longus.	side of
GALL BLADDER	GB 39	Hsüan Chung	3 AUM above malleolus between posterior border of fibula and tendons of peronaeus longus and brevis.	surgery only.
SPLEEN	Sp 6	San Yin Chiao	3 AUM[1] above tip of medial malleolus, just posterior to tibial border.	Electrical stimulation.
BLADDER	B 59	Fu Yang	3 AUM superior to lateral malleolus, posterior to fibula.	
GALL BLADDER	GB 36	Wai Ch'iu	7 AUM superior to lateral malleolus, posterior to fibula.	
STOMACH	St 40	Feng Lung	8 AUM below knee crease, lateral to fibula.	

[1] Note some Western authorities give this as 4 AUM.

8

Acupuncture and Addiction

Addiction to, or dependence upon, any substance can be physiological or psychological, or more likely a combination of both. The precise mechanisms of addiction are not yet clear. Some forms appear to depend upon the biochemical make up of the individual, as well as particular personality traits. Whether these traits are inborn or acquired is the subject of debate. The connection between allergy and addictions, or cravings, is becoming clearer. Some workers maintain that excessive craving for any substance indicates an allergic condition in relation to that substance.[1] Psychological dependence upon a substance is part of the picture in most addictions and must be taken into account in attempting to break habits.

Acupuncture's ability to minimize withdrawal symptoms combined with its undoubted psychologically supportive role makes it a useful aid in such an endeavour. The degree of success in its application varies with the type of addiction. The greatest success is claimed for Acupuncture's use in reducing the withdrawal symptoms from alcohol, cigarettes, narcotics and food (obesity).[2] It has less effect in producing similar benefits in cases of addiction to such drugs as amphetamines, certain tranquillizers, barbiturates and cortisone derivatives.

Since the discovery, in 1975, of naturally occurring analgesic substances, in the body (endorphins and enkephalins) part of the mechanism by which acupuncture assists in relieving the withdrawal symptoms of addiction has become clearer. If, as has been shown,[3] the body contains morphine receptors then it must be capable of producing its own compounds with morphine-like effects. Endorphins have been found in many body tissues[4] such as the brain, CSF, Pituitary gland, adrenal glands, gastro-intestinal system and circulating in the blood. These substances are not identical but are all endogenous peptides, production of which is capable of being stimulated by acupuncture. It is hypothesized that one of the effects of

[1] Philpott, William H., M.D., and Kalita, Dwight K., Ph.D., *Brain Allergies. The Psychonutrient Connection*, Keats Publishing Inc., 1980.

[2] Wexu, Mario, *A Modern Guide to Ear Acupuncture*, ASI Publishers Inc., New York, 1975 (available through Thorsons).

Wensel, Louise O., M.D., *Acupuncture in Medical Practice*, Reston Publishing Co., 1980.

[3] Pomeranz, B., Cheng, R. and Law, P., 'Acupuncture and Responses to Noxious Stimuli: Pituitary Implications', *Experimental Neurology*, 1977, No. 54, pp 172-8.

[4] Snyder, Solomon, 'The Opiate Receptor and Morphine-like Peptides in the Brain', *American Journal of Psychiatry*, June 1976, pp 645-52.

Sjolund, B., Terenius L. and Eriksson, M., 'Increased Cerebro-spinal Fluid Levels of Endorphin After Electro Acupuncture', *Acta Physiologica Scandinavica*, July 1977, p 382.

Goldstein, A., 'Opiod Peptides (Endorphins) in Pituitary and Brain', *Science*, 1976, No. 193, p 1081.

Pert, C., Pert, A. and Tallman, J., 'Isolation of a Novel Opiate Analgesic from Human Blood', *Proceedings of National Academy of Science, U.S.A.*, 1976, No. 73, pp 2226-30.

acupuncture on the addict is to reduce his need for the exogenous drug by allowing his body to produce its own. This helps the breaking of the habit of use, be it smoking, drinking, injecting or swallowing the substance. This does not account entirely for the benefits of acupuncture, but it is a rational starting point. The well established calming or sedating effect of acupuncture, together with the psychologically important supportive[5] and tangible nature of acupuncture treatment is also of importance.

In all cases of addiction it is desirable that there also be some degree of psychotherapy (group therapy, counselling etc.) as well as specific dietary advice, since most addicts suffer from a degree of malnutrition and vitamin and mineral imbalance.

Acupuncture is never a substitute for either of these two essential elements, in attempting to aid the breaking of an addiction. It is, however, an aid to such an effort, especially in reinforcing the individual's own will to succeed, and in often dramatically reducing the distressing symptoms of withdrawal.

The amount of treatment required will vary from one individual to another and with the type of addiction, and some guidance will be given in this regard in the text.

The feeling of well-being which many addicts derive from acupuncture greatly enhances the undoubted effort they are making. The physical withdrawal symptoms of all addictions can be extremely distressing. Ranging from tremors, prostration, cramps, vomiting, sweating, hallucinations etc., to coma and even death. It is therefore of the utmost importance that expert professional supervision be available in attempting to break drug or alcohol dependence. In tobacco addiction, and in cases of habitual overeating, symptoms of withdrawal, whilst unpleasant, will not be as marked. In such cases some degree of supervision, whilst desirable, is not essential.

After breaking any addictive habit there may be a need for periodic maintenance treatment. Guidance will be given in the text.

The application of the acupuncture treatment of addiction falls into the following catagories:
1.   Alcoholism.
2.   Drug addiction.
3.   Food addiction (compulsive eating, obesity etc).
4.   Tobacco addiction.

ALCOHOLISM

It is not suggested that acupuncture alone will enable the individual to break the addiction to alcohol. Due regard must be paid to the physical and psychological needs of the addict. In practice this means paying attention to improving the nutritional status. Many alcoholics are severely malnourished, often exhibiting evidence of hypoglycaemia as well as gross deficiency in, among others Vitamin B_1,

[5] Bresher, David and Koening, Richard, 'Three Essential Factors in Effective Acupuncture', American Journal of Chinese Medicine, 1976, No. 4, pp81-6.

B_3 and B_6. A balanced dietary pattern generous in protein and low in refined carbohydrates is the usual choice, together with supplementation of essential nutrients. The diet should also avoid substances such as caffeine which have a provocative effect on the hypoglycaemic state which usually accompanies alcoholism. Thus tea, coffee, chocolate, cocoa, cola drinks and other caffeine-rich substances should be avoided. Clinical ecologists suggest also removing from the diet foods used in the production of alcoholic beverages such as malt, corn, wheat, barley etc. during withdrawal stage[6].

Counselling and psychotherapy are also key factors in rehabilitating the alcohol dependent person. The short term use of drugs is often advocated in the treatment but this can result in dependence being switched to the substitute, as well of course as a new crop of undesirable side-effects becoming a possibility.

It is in the role of a pacifier during the withdrawal stage that acupuncture comes into its own. In extreme cases these symptoms can be so severe as to endanger life itself, and they must not be minimized. For this reason alone, if acupuncture is to be used to modify, and allay, withdrawal symptoms it must be readily available in the early stages; say the first week. During this time acupuncture treatment can relieve anxiety and withdrawal symptoms, promote a sense of well-being and help to balance the disturbed metabolism of the individual.

For the first five to seven days there should be daily treatment, and in cases where withdrawal reactions are severe treatment should be given twice daily.

Ten to twelve treatments at these close intervals will usually provide sufficient support to enable the initial crisis to be coped with without drugs and with reasonable comfort. Needless to say the nutritional and psychological approach should be concurrent with the acupuncture treatment.

Because of the need for treatments at such close intervals it is frequently suggested that the first week or so of withdrawal should be conducted in an institutional environment. This is ideal but not always practical and many suggest that good results are obtained in an outpatient setting.[7]. The important criterion would seem to be the need for easy access to acupuncture treatment in case of exacerbation of withdrawal symptoms, *at any time*, during the initial week to ten days. As soon as there is a noticeable improvement in the individual's subjective and objective condition, the treatment should be spread to alternate days and thereafter, as the condition continues to stabilize, spread further apart.

In some cases a degree of stability is achieved after only three or four treatments. In some cases no subsequent maintenance acupuncture therapy is needed, once the withdrawal stage is passed, but in others regular 'booster' treatment at weekly, monthly or at greater intervals, seems to assist in the maintenance of the sober state. Whether this is purely a psychological reinforcement of the effort to avoid alcohol, or a biochemical or metabolic balancing effect, is not clear. What is certain is that it is free of side effects.

[6]Dickey, Lawrence, M.D., (Editor) *Clinical Ecology*, Charles C. Thomas, U.S.A., 1976.
[7]See Footnote [2] on page 12.

Choice of Points

A combination of body and ear points are used bilaterally. Points may be selected according to the particular symptoms of withdrawal and they may be varied from treatment to treatment according to variations in such symptoms.

The following ear points are indicated for alcoholism:

Brain
Liver   One or two of these (bilaterally) at each
Kidney   treatment. Select according to degree of
Spleen   sensitivity to pressure.
Stomach

The following are body points most frequently employed in treating withdrawal symptoms from alcohol addiction:

Stomach	6, 8, 36, 37
Governor Vessel	20, 26
Gall Bladder	20 and 34
Bladder	10 and 54
Large Intestine	4 and 11, 18
Lung	7
Spleen	1 and 6, 4
Kidney	1, 3, 7
Circulation	4 and 6
Vessel of Conception	4, 22
Heart	7

Where points are coupled by the word 'and' they may both be used (bilaterally) to enhance the effect.

Apart from selection according to sensitivity, the symptom picture which can assist in selection from the body points listed above are as follows:

Insomnia, abdominal distension confusion, disorientation	Sp1, K1, St36, LI4
Sweating profusely	LI4, K7
Loss of appetite	CV22, C6, LI4, LI18
Excessive salivation	GV26, ST6, LI4, St40
Extreme agitation	Sp6, K3, K1, H7, GV26, C6, LI4
Diarrhoea	St37, B10
Palpitation	C6, C4, H7
Disorientation and dizziness	GV20, GB20, GB34
Vomiting and Nausea	C6, St36, K1
Watering eyes	St8
Acid Stomach, dyspepsia	St36, Sp4
Cystitis	B54
Exhaustion	CV4, St36
Headache	Lu7, St8, K1, GB20, GV20, LI4
Headache	(see also pages 99 to 109)

164

It is suggested that one or two ear points are used at each treatment as well as one of the formula listed above. All these should be employed bilaterally. Points which palpate as particularly tender should be electrically sedated for twenty minutes or more after needles have been inserted.

Patient's Reaction to Treatments

All or some of the following may be reported after a period of electrical stimulation of selected needles.

A feeling of ease.

Reduction of previous symptoms.

Dryness of nose or mouth or eyes.

Feeling of comfortable warmth.

Desire for a warm drink.

Breathing easier.

Urge to urinate.

At this point electrical stimulation should cease and the patient encouraged to relax and sleep if possible.

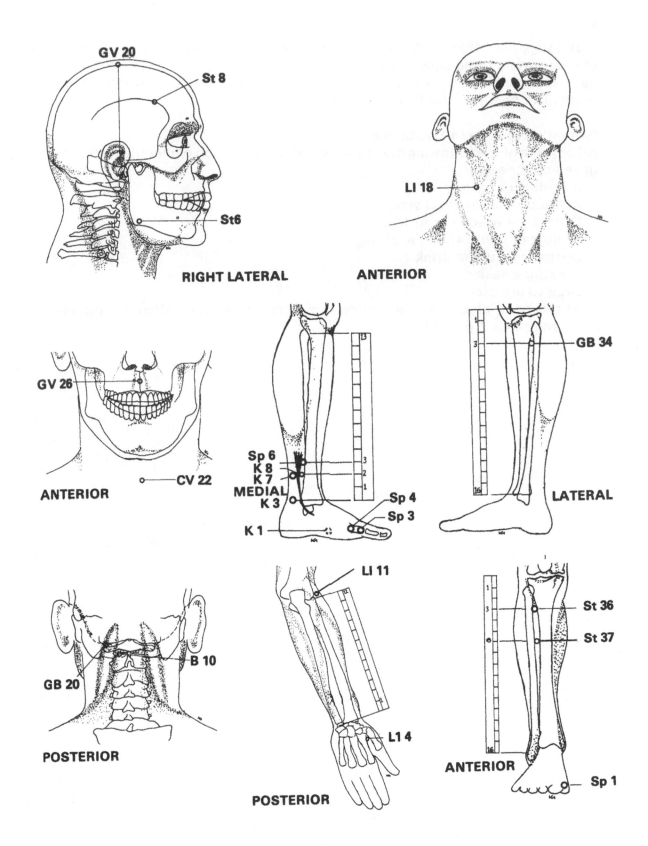

GV 20

St 8

St6

RIGHT LATERAL

LI 18

ANTERIOR

GV 26

CV 22

ANTERIOR

Sp 6
K 8
K 7
MEDIAL
K 3

Sp 4
Sp 3

K 1

GB 34

LATERAL

GB 20

B 10

POSTERIOR

LI 11

L1 4

POSTERIOR

St 36

St 37

ANTERIOR

Sp 1

ALCOHOLISM

Meridian	Point Ref	Chinese Name	Anatomical Position	Depth of Insertion (inches)	Notes
STOMACH	St 6	Chia Ch'ê	At angle of jaw between insertions of masseter muscle.	1	Towards corner of mouth or perpendicularly.
	St 8	T'ou Wei	On a line between external auditory meatus and midline of anterior hairline, just anterior to fronto-pariatal suture.	¼	
	St 36	(Tsu) San Li	3 AUM below depression lateral to patella, one finger's width lateral to crest of tibia.	1-1½	Insert obliquely medially.
	St 37	Ch'eng Shan	8 AUM below knee crease inferior to belly of gastro-cnemeus.	1-1½	
GOVERNOR VESSEL	GV 20	Pai Hui	On midline of skull 7 AUM proximal to posterior hairline.	¼	
	GV 26	Shui Kou	Median line of face, below nose; centre of philtrum.	¼	
GALL BLADDER	GB 20	Feng Ch'ih	Between depression inferior to occipital protuberance and the mastoid bone.	¾	
	GB 34	Yang Ling Ch'üan	In the depression antero-inferior to small head of fibula.	1¼	
LARGE INTESTINE	LI 4	Ho Ku	Dorsal surface of hand in angle of first 2 metacarpals	1	Strong stimulation.
	LI 11	Ch'u Ch'ih	Lateral aspect of elbow crease between lateral epicondyle and edge of elbow fold.	1	
	LI 18	Fu Tu	3 AUM lateral to thyroid cartilage, between sternal head and clavicular head of sterno-cleido mastoid muscle.	¾	
SPLEEN	Sp 1	Yin Pai	Just proximal to angle of root of nail of great toe medial aspect.	¼	
	Sp 4	Kung Sun	Medial aspect of foot 1 AUM proximal to articulation of metatarsal and phalange of great toe.	¾	
	Sp 6	San Yin Chiao	3 AUM above tip of internal malleolus, posterior to tibial border.	½ to 1½	

167

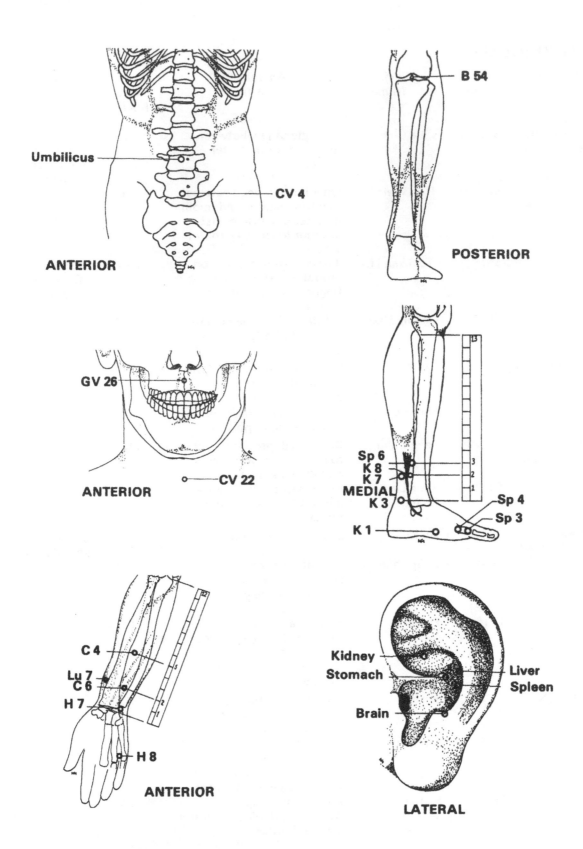

ANTERIOR

Umbilicus

CV 4

POSTERIOR

B 54

GV 26

ANTERIOR

CV 22

MEDIAL

Sp 6
K 8
K 7
K 3
K 1
Sp 4
Sp 3

C 4
Lu 7
C 6
H 7
H 8

ANTERIOR

LATERAL

Kidney
Stomach
Brain
Liver
Spleen

ALCOHOLISM (contd.)

Meridian	Point Ref	Chinese Name	Anatomical Position	Depth of Insertion (inches)	Notes
LUNG	L 7	Lieh Ch'üeh	1½ AUM proximal to transverse wrist crease, above styloid process of radius.	½	Insert needle obliquely upwards.
KIDNEY	K 1	Yung Ch'üan	Centre of sole of foot in crease formed when toes are flexed.	¾	
	K 3	T'ai Ch'i	Internal aspect of foot ½ AUM posterior to malleolus.	½	
	K 7	Fu Liu	Internal aspect of leg 3 AUM above internal malleolus, behind flexor digitorum longus.	½	
CIRCULA-TION	C 4	Ch'i Men	Anterior surface of forearm between ulna and radius, 5 AUM proximal to wrist crease.	½	
	C 6	Nei Kuan	2 AUM above wrist crease between tendons of palmaris longus and flexor carpi radialis.	¾	
CONCEP-TION VESSEL	CV 4	Kuan Yüan	On midline, 3 AUM below umbilicus	¾	
	CV 22	T'ien T'u	On the anterior midline 1½ AUM proximal to superior edge of supra-sternal notch.	¼	
HEART	H 7	Shen Men	Ulna aspect of wrist on proximal border of pisiform bone, in a depression.	½	
BLADDER	B 10˙	T'ien Chu	Posterior neck. 1½ AUM lateral to midline level with interspace between 1st and 2nd cervical vertebrae.	¾	
	B 54	Wei Chung	Exact centre of popliteal crease.	¾-1½	

Auricular Points

KIDNEY POINT	Upper portion cavum conchae.
ABDOMEN/STOMACH POINT	Upper portion cavum conchae.
LIVER POINT	Right auricle, postero-inferior aspect cymba-conchae.
SPLEEN POINT	Left auricle, postero-inferior aspect cymba-conchae.
BRAIN POINT	Lateral aspect Antitragus.

TOBACCO ADDICTION

As with alcoholism it is desirable that there be a complementary nutritional and psychological programme to accompany acupuncture therapy. The individual should be strongly motivated and should have analysed the reasons which lie behind the addiction or habit. These can range from a need for stimulation; to a belief in the apparent relaxing effect; to a pleasure in the ritual of the act; to pure habit and, in some cases, to actual physical addiction. Counselling and support and understanding will help enormously to enhance the individuals motivation. Acupuncture can reinforce this as well as reducing the actual craving, and the withdrawal symptoms.

Nutritional advice: The individual should, for the first two weeks of stopping smoking, avoid highly spiced or seasoned meals and stop tea, coffee and alcohol consumption. This helps to break habitual relationships which often exist between these foods and beverages, and smoking. The following supplements are suggested for at least the first month to six weeks of the non-smoking period: Vitamin A 15,000 i.u., Vitamin E 400 i.u., Niacinamide 500mg. Calcium Pantothenate 500mg, 1 high potency B complex (to contain at least 50mg each of thiamin, riboflavin and pyridoxine), Vitamin B_{12} 500 micrograms.

Choice of Points

Ear Points: Lower jaw, Upper jaw, Shenmen, Lung, Pharynx, Abdomen, Kidney, Int. Nose.

Body Points: H7, C6, GV24, L4, 5, and 7, LI4 and 13, St36 and 40, Sp8.

Choose one of two pairs of ear points, according to sensitivity, as well as one or two body points according to symptoms e.g:

Headache	LI4, GV24, L7
Dizziness	St40, GV24
Restlessness and agitation	C6, LI4, H7, GV24
Insomnia	C6, H7, GV24
Indigestion, activity, nausea	St36, C6, Sp8
Cough	St40, L4, L5
Tight chest	C6, L7, L4, LI13
Runny nose	GV24

Repeated treatments, daily at first or at least three times in the first week of stopping smoking, are indicated. The recent practice of inserting a staple or press needle, and leaving it in situ for days or weeks. so that the patient can manipulate it at times of craving and or during withdrawal symptoms, is not as effective, and holds the potential for localized infection of the external ear and subsequent scar tissue formation in the area.

As in alcoholism one or two bilateral ear points as well as one or two body points should be electrically stimulated at each treatment, for a minimum of twenty minutes. Ideally some subjective reaction from the patient (see *patient's reaction to treatment* page 165) should take place. At the very least a relative sense of calmness and well being should result. Counselling and encouragement should be forthcoming. The patient should be told that as a result of the treatment the craving will tend to diminish and the unpleasant side effects be moderated, but that both these aspects will still be noticed, and that their own determination to achieve success is still called for. If total reliance is placed upon the treatment by the patient, without personal effort, then success is less likely.

Up to ten treatments over a three or four week period may be needed to break the habit.

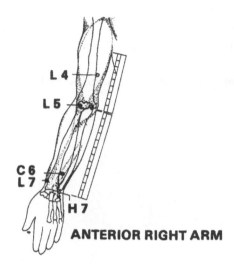

ANTERIOR RIGHT ARM

L 4
L 5
C 6
L 7
H 7

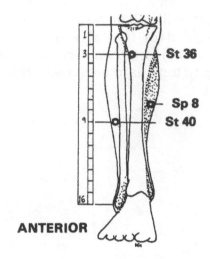

ANTERIOR

St 36
Sp 8
St 40

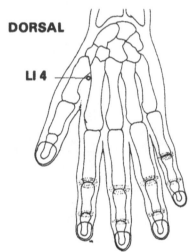

DORSAL

LI 4

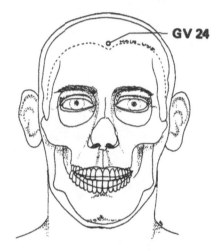

GV 24

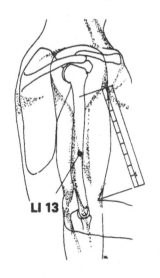

LI 13

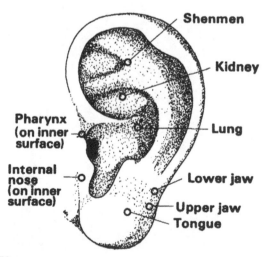

Shenmen

Kidney

Pharynx
(on inner
surface)

Lung

Internal
nose
(on inner
surface)

Lower jaw

Upper jaw
Tongue

TOBACCO ADDICTION

Meridian	Point Ref	Chinese Name	Anatomical Position	Depth of Insertion (inches)	Notes
LUNG	L 4	Hsieh Pai	5 AUM proximal to elbow crease on median line of biceps.	¾	
	L 5	Ch'ih Chih	On.elbow crease lateral to biceps tendon.	¾	
	L 7	Lieh Ch'üeh	Anterior surface of forearm lateral to radial artery 2 AUM proximal to wrist crease.	½	
HEART	H 7	Shen Men	Ulnar aspect of wrist on proximal border of pisiform bone, in a depression.	½	
CIRCU-LATION	C 6	Nei Kuan	2 AUM above wrist crease between tendons of palmaris longus and flexor carpi radialis.	¾	
GOVERNOR VESSEL	GV 24	Shent'ing	On midline ½ AUM cephalid to anterior hairline.	½	Obliquely
SPLEEN	Sp 8	Ti'Chi	On posterior border of tibia on internal aspect of leg 9 AUM superior to internal malleolus.	1	
STOMACH	St 36	(Tsu) San Li	3 AUM below depression lateral to patella, one finger's width lateral to crest of fibia.	1-1½	Insert obliquely
	St 40	Feng Lung	Lateral surface of leg 8 AUM inferior to knee crease, posterior to tibialis anterior.	1	
LARGE INTESTINE	LI 4	Ho Ku	Dorsal surface of hand in angle of first two metacarpals.	1	
	LI 13	(Yang) Wu Li	Lateral surface of arm 3½ AUM proximal to elbow crease.	½	

Auricular Points

PHARYNX POINT — Inner surface of tragus, opposite external auditory meatus.

INTERNAL NOSE POINT — Inner surface of Tragus, inferior to pharynx point.

TONGUE POINT — Central Ear Lobe.

UPPER JAW POINTS ⎤
LOWER JAW POINTS ⎦ — In posterior region of ear lobe, locate by pressure and sensitivity.

LUNG POINT — Centre of cavum conchae.

KIDNEY POINT — Upper portion of cávum conchae.

SHENMEN POINT — In inferior corner of bifurcating point of antihelix.

DRUG ADDICTION

It must be emphasized at the outset that drug addiction should be treated only under expert supervision, preferably institutionally. Further, it should only be attempted if there is an expert knowledge of the potential effects of withdrawal of the particular drug(s), and whether this should be a sudden or gradual process. Unless there is a supportive, stress-free, environment, coupled with counselling and psychotherapy, there is unlikely to be a succesful outcome to such an effort.

Acupuncture does provide a unique method of enhancing the process of breaking such an addiction. It is suggested that particular attention also be paid to nutrition. A wholefood high protein diet, is often the most suitable, coupled with a supply of high potency multimineral and multivitamin supplements. The intake of B vitamins should be in mega-doses for some weeks (e.g. 500mg daily niacinamide, 100mg daily pyridoxine) and vitamin C should be taken in doses of several grams daily.

Treatment should be daily during the initial withdrawal stage, and if symptoms indicate it, twice daily. Once this acute stage is passed the treatments should be reduced to three, then two times, weekly, with a possible weekly 'booster' for some months, being helpful for long-term addicts.

Each treatment should employ a selection of ear and body points, approximately eight to ten needles being used at each treatment. Selection of ear points is by sensitivity to pressure. Body points are chosen according to their known effect on particular symptom patterns. Some of the needles should be electrically stimulated (saw-tooth or square wave pulsating current, 30 to 100 micro-amperes).

Treatments are reduced to every second or third day as soon as marked improvement becomes apparent.

Individual treatment can last from twenty to fifty minutes. Electrical stimulation being modified to the patient's tolerance. The sensation should not be unpleasant but should be slightly more than mild. If the patient reports a sensation of warmth and ease of breathing, or a dryness of eyes, mouth or nose, or a marked urge to urinate, or a desire for a warm drink, during treatment then it is usually time to terminate that session. The patient should be encouraged to take gentle outdoor exercise and to sleep as much as possible.

Choice of Points
Ear Points: Brain, Lung, Liver, Abdomen.
Body Points: LI4, St8, 15, 25 and 40; CV10, 12, 13 and 14; GV20; GB20 and 34; K1; C6 and 7; Sp1 and 6; H7; L7; SI3; TH5, 6.

Selection of body points according to symptoms:

Restlessness and agitation	C6, LI4, H7, Sp 1 + 6, CV14, GV 20, GB20 + 34, K1
Nausea	St36, C6, K1
Headache	LI4, L7, K1, GV20, GB20 + 34, S13 TH5, St8
Exhaustion	St36
Vomiting	St36, K1, C6 + 7, CV12, 13, 14
Bowel involvement (diarrhoea, distension etc.)	St36, CV10, 12, 13, 14, C6, Sp6, St 25 + 40
Chills	GB 20 + 34, TH5, TH6
Light sensitivity	St8
Insomnia	C 6 + 7 H7
Eyes watering	St8
Palpitation	C6 + 7, CV14
Extreme neck tension	SI3, St40
Night Sweats	St3
Frequency of urination or retention	Sp6
Sore throat	TH6

It is worth noting that the suggestion that acupuncture's role is largely a psychologically supportive one is found to be untrue. Whilst this is undoubtedly a factor in its effectiveness, there tends to be a high degree of scepticism and disbelief on the part of many drug users regarding its ability to help them through withdrawal, especially if the individual has made previously unassisted attempts. Their surprise and gratitude at its value is in sharp contrast to their often initial reluctant, and even hostile attitude towards it.

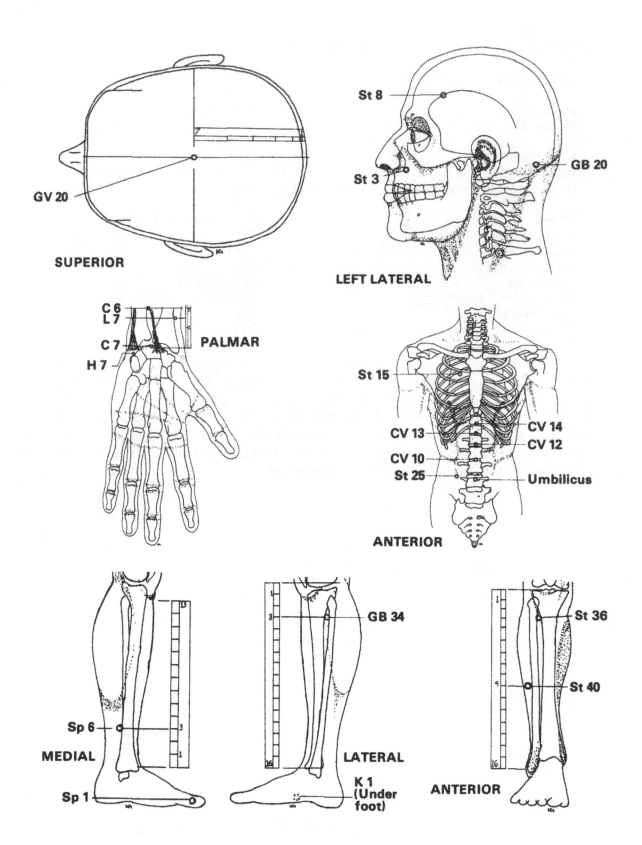

SUPERIOR

LEFT LATERAL

St 8

St 3

GB 20

PALMAR

C 6
L 7

C 7

H 7

St 15

CV 13

CV 14

CV 12

CV 10

St 25

Umbilicus

ANTERIOR

Sp 6

MEDIAL

Sp 1

GB 34

LATERAL

K 1
(Under
foot)

St 36

St 40

ANTERIOR

DRUG ADDICTION

Meridian	Point Ref	Chinese Name	Anatomical Position	Depth of Insertion (inches)	Notes
GOVERNOR VESSEL	GV 20	Pai Hui	On midline of skull 7 AUM cephalid to posterior hairline.	1¼	
CONCEP-TION VESSEL	CV 10	Hsia Kuan	On midline of abdomen 2 AUM above umbilicus.	1	Perpendicularly.
	CV 12	Chung Kuan	Midpoint between umbilicus and xyphoid process, 4 AUM above umbilicus.	1	Perpendicularly.
	CV 13	Shang Kuan	5 AUM above umbilicus.	1	Perpendicularly.
	CV 14	Chu Ch'üeh	6 AUM above umbilicus.	1	Obliquely downwards.
GALL BLADDER	GB 20	Fêng Ch'ih	Between depression inferior to occipital protuberance and mastoid bone.	¾	
	GB 34	Yang Ling Ch'üan	In depression antero-inferior to small head of fibula.	1¼	
STOMACH	St 3	Chü Liao	Directly below Stomach 2 at level of lower end of ala nasi, lateral to groove.	½	
	St 8	T'ou Wei	On a line between external auditory meatus and midline of anterior hairline, just anterior to fronto-parietal suture.	¼	
	St 15	Wu I	Directly above nipple in 2nd costal interspace.	½	
	St 25	Tien Ch'u	2 AUM lateral to umbilicus.	¾	Perpendicularly.
	St 36	(Tsu) San Li	3 AUM below depression lateral to patella, one finger's width lateral to crest of tibia.	1-1½	Insert obliquely medially.
	St 40	Feng Lung	Lateral surface of leg, 8 AUM inferior to knee crease level, posterior to tibialis anterior.	1	
KIDNEY	K 1	Yung Ch'üan	Centre of sole of foot, in crease formed when toes are flexed.	¾	
SPLEEN	Sp 1	Yin Pai	Just proximal to angle of root of nail of great toe, medial aspect.	¼	
	Sp 6	San Yin Chiao	3 AUM above tip of internal malleolus posterior to tibial border.	½ to 1½	
CIRCULA-TION	C 6	Nei Kuan	2 AUM above wrist crease between tendons of palmaris longus and flexor carpi radialis.	¾	

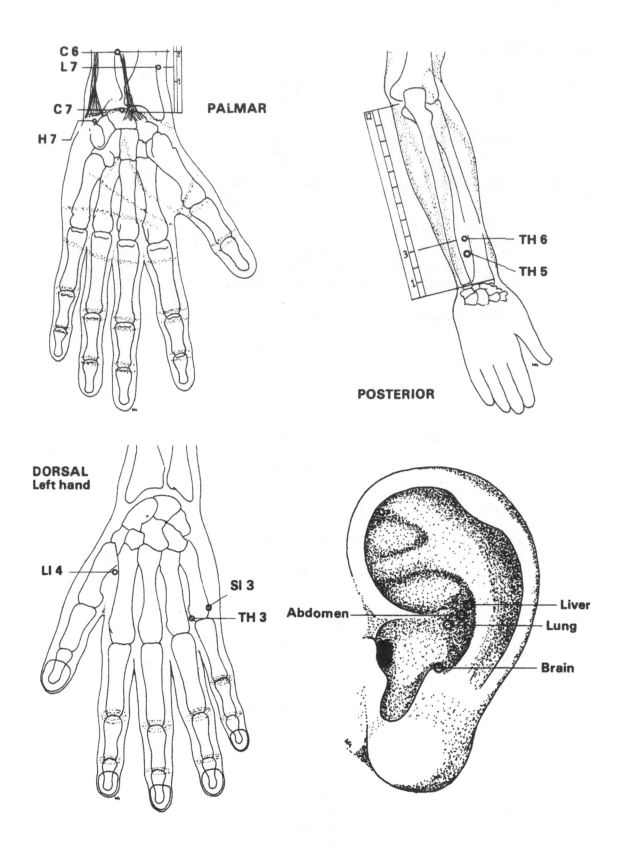

PALMAR

C 6
L 7
C 7
H 7

POSTERIOR

TH 6
TH 5

DORSAL
Left hand

LI 4

SI 3
TH 3

Abdomen

Liver
Lung

Brain

178

DRUG ADDICTION (contd.)

Meridian	Point Ref	Chinese Name	Anatomical Position	Depth of Insertion (inches)	Notes
	C 7	Ta Ling	Midpoint of transverse wrist crease.	¼	
LUNG	L 7	Lieh Ch'üeh	1½ AUM proximal to transverse wrist crease, above styloid process of radius.	½	Obliquely upwards.
HEART	H 7	Shen Men	Ulna aspect of wrist on proximal border of pisiform bone, in a depression.	½	
LARGE INTESTINE	LI 4	Ho Ku	Dorsal surface of hand in angle of first 2 metacarpals.	1	
TRIPLE HEATER	TH 3	Chung Chu	Dorsal surface of hand posterior to and between 4th and 5th metacarpal bones, in a depression.	½	Perpendicularly.
	TH 5	Wai Kuan	2 AUM proximal to wrist crease on dorsal surface, between radius and ulna.	½	Perpendicularly.
	TH 6	Chih Kou	1 AUM above TH5 (Wai Kuan).	¾	Perpendicularly.
SMALL INTESTINE	SI 3	Hou Ch'i	Just proximal to metacarpo-phalangeal articulation of little finger.	¼	

Auricular Points

LIVER POINT	Right auricle, posterio-inferior aspect cymba-conchae.
STOMACH POINT	Upper portion cavum conchae.
LUNG POINT	Centre of cavum conchae.
BRAIN POINT	Lateral aspect anti-tragus.

FOOD ADDICTION (AND OBESITY)

Diet and exercise are fundamental to weight reduction. Acupuncture can assist by (a) promoting a sense or well being which reduces compulsive eating; (b) improving general metabolism; (c) increasing willpower and determination. The points will depend upon the underlying causes of the problem and these will be indicated in the formulae below.

Choice of Points

Ear points may be selected from the following, according to sensitivity and general indications:

If food addiction results from personality or emotional causes:

Brain; Occiput; Shenmen; Stomach; Lungs; Subcortex.

It is suggested that one point and Shenmen be utilized at each treatment (bilaterally) as well as appropriate body points.

If obesity is due to hormonal imbalance:

Hormone; Brain; Testicle/ovary; Sympathy. Thyroid; Hypothalamus (Nogier).

If due to malabsorption and/or liver dysfunction:

Liver; Gall Bladder; Abdomen; Occiput; Metabolism (Nogier); Zero point (Nogier).

For general weight control from above, or any of the following, according to sensitivity:

Colon; Small Intestine; Kidney.

Body Points:

CV4, 6, 8, 10; St25 and 36; Sp6 + 9; TH6; C6 + 9.

The choice of these will depend upon the general assessment of the patient's condition and the indications of the body points mentioned. The following brief information will assist in this choice.

Abdominal Distension	CV4, 6, 8, Sp 6 + 9 St 36.
Irregular (loose) bowels	CV4, 8(+ 11), Sp6, St25.
Oedema	CV6 + 11(+ 8), Sp6 + 9.
Gastric and digestive disturbance.	St36, CV11 (+ 8), C6 + 9.
Agitation	C6 + 9.
Nervous exhaustion (and general tonic effect)	Sp6, St36, CV4.
Constipation	St25 + 36, TH6.
Hiccough	C6.
Vomiting	C6 + 9.
Irregular Menstruation	Sp6 + 9, CV4 + 6.
Bladder Symptoms (Frequency or urine retention)	Sp6.

A series of ten or more treatments at intervals of four to seven days together with general guidance, counselling and specific dietary advice, should result in reduction in weight as well as diminution of compulsive eating habits.

The use of residual staples or press point needles is not recommended due to the danger of local infection. Electrical stimulation of ear and body points enhances the effect of treatment but is not essential.

N.B. It should be noted that food addiction, as construed in this work, is a generalized condition, i.e. habitually eating too much, rather than cravings for particular foods which would probably indicate a masked allergic response to that food.

Philpot[8] characterizes addiction in the following manner: 'Initial relief or partial relief (of symptoms) on exposure (ingestion, inhalation etc.) and the emergence of delayed reactions, which can again be relieved by exposure.' It is certainly possible for acupuncture to assist in the normalizing of such specific addiction allergic responses of this kind (alcohol and tobacco addiction are often examples of this). However, in the food field, there are 'families' of foods (e.g. cereals) which should be avoided at such times, and a knowledge of clinical ecology methods, and rotation diets would be helpful in their treatment.

[8] See Footnote 1 on page 161.

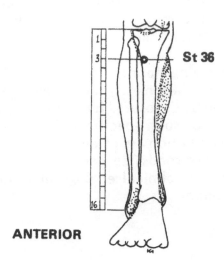

St 36

ANTERIOR

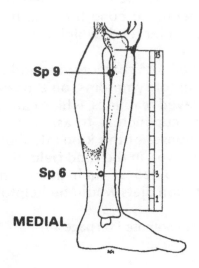

Sp 9

Sp 6

MEDIAL

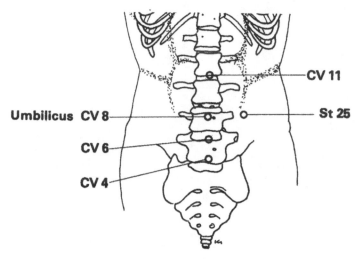

CV 11

Umbilicus CV 8

St 25

CV 6

CV 4

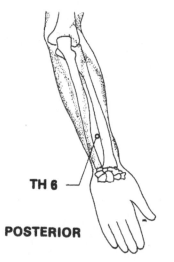

TH 6

POSTERIOR

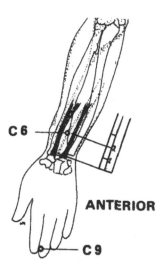

C 6

ANTERIOR

C 9

182

FOOD ADDICTION

Meridian	Point Ref	Chinese Name	Anatomical Position	Depth of Insertion (inches)	Notes
STOMACH	St 25	Tien Ch'u	2 AUM lateral to umbilicus.	¾	Perpendicularly.
	St 36	(Tsu) San Li	3 AUM below depression lateral to patella, one finger's width lateral to crest of tibia.	1-1½	Obliquely medially.
CIRCULA-TION	C 6	Nei Kuan	2 AUM above wrist crease between tendons of palmaris longus and flexor carpi radialis.	¾	
	C 9	Chung Heng	At the midpoint of tip of middle finger.	⅛	
TRIPLE HEATER	TH 6	Chih Kou	3 AUM proximal to wrist crease, on posterior surface of forearm, between radius and ulna.	¾	Perpendicularly.
SPLEEN	Sp 6	San Yin Chiao	3 AUM above tip of internal malleolus posterior to tibial border.	½-1½	
	Sp 9	Yin Ling Ch'üan	In depression on lower border of medial condyle of tibia, level with tibial tuberosity.	1	
CONCEP-TION VESSEL	CV 4	Kuan Yüan	3 AUM below umbilicus on midline.	1	
	CV 6	Ch'i Hai	1½ AUM below umbilicus on midline.	1	
	CV 8	Shen Ch'ueh	In centre of umbilicus.		Needle forbidden use moxibustion only.
	CV 11	Chien Li	3 AUM above umbilicus on midline.	1	

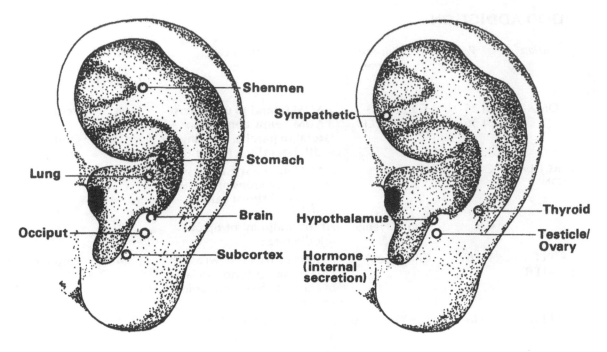

Top left diagram labels:
Shenmen
Sympathetic
Stomach
Lung
Brain
Occiput
Subcortex

LATERAL

Top right diagram labels:
Sympathetic
Thyroid
Hypothalamus
Testicle/Ovary
Hormone (internal secretion)

LATERAL

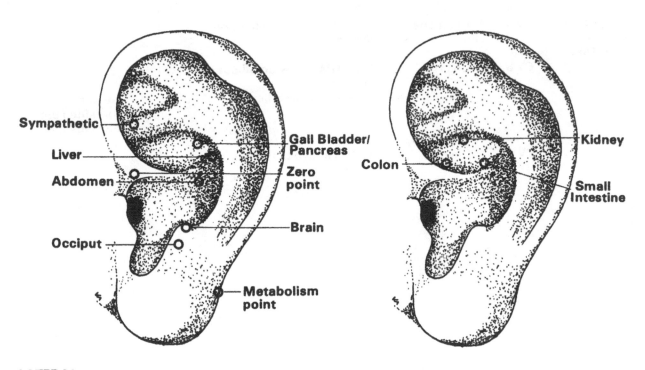

Bottom left diagram labels:
Sympathetic
Gall Bladder/Pancreas
Liver
Zero point
Abdomen
Occiput
Brain
Metabolism point

LATERAL

Bottom right diagram labels:
Kidney
Colon
Small Intestine

LATERAL

FOOD ADDICTION (contd.)

Auricular Points

1. *Personality and Emotional Causes:*

BRAIN POINT	Lateral aspect antitragus.
OCCIPUT POINT	Postero-superior aspect antitragus.
SHENMEN POINT	In inferior corner of bifurcating point of antihelix.
STOMACH POINT	Upper portion cavum conchae.
LUNG POINT	Centre of cavum conchae.
SUBCORTEX POINT	Inferior wall antitragus.

2. *Hormonal Imbalance:*

SYMPATHETIC POINT	In deltoid fossa at junction of infra-antihelix crus and medial border of helix.
HYPOTHALAMUS POINT	At apex of antitragus, on the rim.
HORMONE (INTERNAL SECRETION POINT)	Base of inter-tragic notch.
TESTICLE/OVARY POINT	Medial aspect of inner surface of antitragus.
THYROID POINT	Above posterior auricular sulcus, near the scapha.

3. *Malabsorption:*

ZERO POINT (Nogier)	Root of antihelix in a notch.
SYMPATHETIC POINT	In deltoid fossa at junction of infra-antihelix crus and medial border of helix.
GALL BLADDER/PANCREAS POINTS	Gall bladder, right ear; pancreas, left ear, above foot of crus of helix.
LIVER POINT	Right auricle, postero-inferior aspect cymba-conchae.
ABDOMEN/STOMACH POINTS	Upper portion cavum conchae.
BRAIN POINT	Lateral aspect antitragus.
OCCIPUT POINT	Postero-superior aspect of antitragus.
METABOLISM POINT (Nogier)	Supero-posterior aspect of lobe.

4. *Weight Control:*

COLON POINT	Above crust of helix.
KIDNEY POINT	Upper portion cavum conchae.
SMALL INTESTINE POINT	Superior to crus of helix. Posterior to colon point.

INDEX

BOOKS OF RELATED INTEREST

Soft-Tissue Manipulation
A Practitioner's Guide to the Diagnosis
and Treatment of Soft-Tissue Dysfunction and Reflex Activity
by Leon Chaitow, D.O., N.D.

Is Acupuncture Right for You?
What It Is, Why It Works, and How It Can Help You
by Ruth Lever Kidson

Acupuncture Imaging
Perceiving the Energy Pathways of the Body
by Mark D. Seem, Ph.D., DIPL. AC. (NCAA)

Acupuncture Energetics
A Workbook for Diagnostics and Treatment
by Mark Seem, Ph.D.

The Acupressure Atlas
by Bernard C. Kolster, M.D.,
and Astrid Waskowiak, M.D.

Acupressure Techniques
A Self-Help Guide
by Julian Kenyon, M.D.

Acupressure Taping
The Practice of Acutaping for Chronic Pain and Injuries
by Hans-Ulrich Hecker, M.D.,
and Kay Liebchen, M.D.

Trigger Point Therapy for Myofascial Pain
The Practice of Informed Touch
by Donna Finando, L.Ac., L.M.T.,
and Steven Finando, Ph.D., L.Ac.

Inner Traditions • Bear & Company
P.O. Box 388
Rochester, VT 05767
1-800-246-8648
www.InnerTraditions.com

Or contact your local bookseller